Reading *White Coat Revival* is like getting a defibrillator jolt straight to your soul. The good kind. If you've ever wondered whether God still speaks in the exam room, this book proves He does. Read it and watch burnout lose its power and supernatural become your new life.

— **ED RUSH**, Author *God Talks*, GodTalks.com

White Coat Revival is the clearest roadmap I've found for reclaiming purpose, presence, and truth in the practice of medicine-Marilyn Kaminski delivers what physicians desperately need: a way back to wholeness, calling, and the sacred art of healing. A must-read for any doctor ready to lead with the spirit and the soul rather than survive the system.

— **DR. KEVIN AISTER, D.O.**, Integrative Wellness Physician, Retired Emergency Medicine Physician (37 Years), Scottsdale, Arizona

White Coat Revival returns us to the Great Physician — eyes on Jesus as medical intercessors God designed. He heals; we serve. It invites physicians to pray, align, and act — a worshipful practice of medicine: hope-filled, compassionate, effective.

— **DR. GLORIA TUMBAGA, M.D.**, Physician & Founder, The Institute of Divine Authenticity & Wellness, Temecula, California

As a practicing Chiropractor for over 22 years, I have often wondered how to incorporate my faith in God with my clinical expertise. *White Coat Revival* has opened my eyes in a new way, showing me a path to listen to the very voice of God to help my patients heal on all levels; physically, mentally, spiritually. As health care providers, we do not have to approach patient management alone. We can tap into Jehovah Rapha — the God who Heals and our patients can have supernatural results! This book has taught me how to embrace a partnership with Him and I do not want to practice any other way from now on.

— **DR. JEN WINTON, D.C**, Chiropractor, Activate Lifestyle Clinic, Phoenix, Arizona

Since reading the *White Coat Revival*, I feel like the chains were lifted and I am no longer productivity-led but instead Spirit-led. I get through my workday easier because I partner with God and His amazing power within me! I can't wait for you to experience the same!

— **AMY TIBBITS, PA-C**, Physician Assistant Family Medicine, Mineral Point, Wisconsin

WHITE
COAT
REVIVAL

A simple solution to
empower and restore YOU,
the heart of medicine

WHITE
COAT
REVIVAL

A simple solution to
empower and restore YOU,
the heart of medicine

MARILYN
KAMINSKI

Niche Press
Indianapolis, IN

For permission to reprint portions of this content or bulk purchases, contact Info@WhiteCoatRevival.com

Published by Niche Press; NichePress.com
Indianapolis, IN

Cover design by Joshua Sword

ISBN
Hardcover: 978-1-970329-06-3
Paperback: 978-1-970329-07-0
eBook: 978-1-970329-05-6

Library of Congress Control Number: 2026902392

*This book is dedicated to hearts and souls
who are called into the beautiful role of healing.*

ACCESS YOUR FREE
7 ALIGNMENTS™
SUPPLEMENTAL CONTENT

This book is designed
with **alignment exercises**
so you can pause and
realign to optimize **your
transformation** as you read.

Scan the QR Code below,
enter your email, and I'll
send the additional exercises
and bonus resources straight
to your inbox.

WhiteCoatRevival.com/bonus

TABLE OF CONTENTS

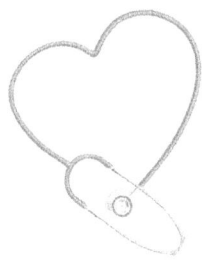

A RETURN TO MEDICINE AS GOD INTENDED

Medicine was never meant to be soulless.

Yet somewhere along the way, buried beneath protocols, productivity metrics, electronic checklists, and relentless time pressure, the heart of healing began to fade. The white coat, once a symbol of sacred trust, compassion, and vocation, has too often become a uniform of exhaustion. Physicians and healers who entered medicine with wonder and calling now find themselves overwhelmed, constrained, and quietly asking a question they scarcely dare to voice:

Is this really all there is?

White Coat Revival was written for that question.

This book is not a rejection of science. It is not an attack on modern medicine. And it is not a call to abandon evidence, rigor, or clinical excellence. Rather, it is an invitation to awaken and recover what has been lost: the integration of science and spirit, skill and soul, knowledge and divine partnership.

As a physician who has practiced at the highest levels of modern medicine, I have seen firsthand the extraordinary power of medical science. I have also witnessed its limitations. No amount of training can replace wisdom. No algorithm can substitute for discernment. And no system — no matter how advanced — can heal the human heart apart from its Creator.

What is missing in medicine today is not intelligence. It is alignment.

White Coat Revival introduces a radical yet profoundly simple truth: The responsibility for healing was never meant to be carried alone. The burden physicians feel — the pressure to fix, solve, and save — was never ours to bear by ourselves. True healing flows through partnership with the Great Physician, who designed the human body and still desires to restore it.

This book is a call to physicians, nurses, clinicians, and all healers to reclaim their rightful places, not as mere technicians of the body, but as *medical intercessors*, standing in the gap between heaven and earth. It is a return to medicine as vocation, not just profession, as ministry, not merely occupation.

Within these pages, you will encounter a framework the author calls **the 7 Alignments**™ — a practical, transformative path that restores harmony between mind and heart, science and Spirit, human effort and divine authority. These alignments do not require changing your specialty, your workplace, or your credentials. They require something far more powerful: a shift in posture from striving to surrender, from isolation to partnership, from burnout to purpose.

This is not about doing more.

It is about aligning differently.

When alignment occurs, something remarkable happens. Peace replaces pressure. Clarity replaces confusion. Compassion deepens. Outcomes change. And the physician — often the most neglected patient in the system — begins to heal.

White Coat Revival is ultimately a love letter from God to His healers, reminding them they are seen, chosen, and still called. It is an invitation to lay down burdens never meant to be carried and to put on a *heavenly white coat* — no longer a garment of exhaustion, but one of authority, humility, and love.

If you feel weary...

If you sense there must be more...

If your heart still longs to heal the way you once imagined...

This book is for you.

The revival begins within.

— **CHAUNCEY W. CRANDALL IV, MD, FACC, FACP,** Author: *Touching Heaven, Raising the Dead, The Simple Heart Cure*

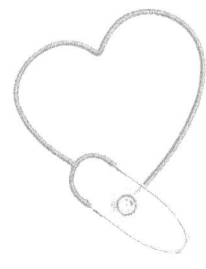

THE QUIET SKILL THAT CHANGES EVERYTHING

If you are reading this, you are one of God's pursued.

Like so many working in healthcare, you started the journey toward your career with a purpose, a heart's desire to help people heal and live prosperous, fulfilling, healthy lives. However, today's medical field holds challenges that often seem to make achieving your heart's desire and God's plan nearly impossible. God wants to change this. He wants to take back the health of His prize creation — the human body — and He wants to do it *through* you by fulfilling the purpose and promises He originally placed in your heart. This starts not by trying to change the industry, but by healing the most important part of the industry — **you**.

Your white coat signifies excellence, authority, and a trust bestowed the moment you enter a patient's presence. Yet in a medical system that has grown technical and transactional, your heart beneath that coat has been muted.

I named this book *White Coat Revival* to reignite the purpose, compassion, and divine calling that make complete healing possible. Whether you are actively practicing, retired, or aspiring to serve others through healing, this message is for you. I encourage all to read this love letter from God because He does indeed love you, and you have a very important role in His divine plan!

With more than two decades of experience in patient care, I know firsthand the challenges you face when trying to love and serve your patients' true needs while navigating the demands of the medical industry. When faced with this struggle, I prayed for answers. **Then, in 2024, God answered my prayers with a series of visions, dreams, and revelations to share with you.**

Nearly every solution that gets incorporated into the medical world is designed to boost patient outcomes or streamline administrative efficiency. You're offered more training, more data, more systems — yet almost nothing speaks to *you:* your heart, your mind, your calling, your spiritual well-being. This book is different. It is a solution for the healer — the person God created you to be — restoring your wholeness so you can flourish and, in turn, see patient outcomes multiply far beyond what the current system alone can produce.

God desires your work to be simple, easy, and light; fulfilling and free from burden and from the many chains that encompass the current medical system. He desires for heaven to come down here on earth. He seeks to heal disease, illness, injury, and infirmities through a partnership combining His divine wisdom with your extraordinary knowledge. He is chasing you down with favor, goodness, grace, and mercy to align your God-given purpose back to His, creating a working relationship through which His light, His love, and His hope flow through you to your patient.

Though you may not realize it, over the years, a disconnect has formed between your mind and your heart.

You carry the responsibility to heal on your own — a burden grounded in your mind — yet your heart longs for something more: love, respect, and tangible evidence of God's promises as a return for the sacrifices you've made.

As a child of God who was called to the vocation of medicine, you have authority to heal the sick and show God's love and magnificent power to the world. This authority needs to be unleashed!

Accept this book as an invitation to activate the authority of Christ. This authority *within you* works through your obedience to the healing calling and in partnership with God through His Holy Spirit.

Within these pages, I will walk you through a transformational process called the 7 Alignments™. This process positions you with a powerful approach utilizing both science and the Holy Spirit to become the healer you were called to be. I introduce this approach as a Medical Intercessor.

A Medical Intercessor has a calling beyond higher education, which is about the inner workings of the human body. Instead, a Medical Intercessor operates as a medically trained healer who stands in the gap (Ezekiel 22:30, NIV) between God and their patients, serving as a conduit for His love and healing. To pour this divine love and healing out for your patients as a Medical Intercessor, you must be fully aligned with and able to attune to the mind of Christ within you.

Using this 7 Alignments framework with the ViaRayma™ practitioners, I and others have experienced miraculous patient outcomes. In this book, you will read about some of those experiences.

More than anything, this book offers a mindset transformation to align your own mind with the mind of Christ. **This is the quiet skill that changes everything about how you approach healing your patient.**

Implementing the 7 Alignments will allow you to operate from your own heart and mind in a way that's 100 percent aligned with God. Because Christ dwells in you, His authority and God's will can flow through you with the help and energy of the Holy Spirit. You will learn to be still and know, working within a parasympathetic nervous system state and using both sides of your brain to approach your patient's healing in a balanced, unified way. You will see what a huge difference that single change actually makes for your patient and you.

In fact, the majority of what I teach you in this book and throughout my courses will work in the background of your patient interactions. Your patient may not even realize you are connecting with the Great Physician unless God directs you to reveal that or the patient asks for prayer. And, if we get an invitation from our patient to pray with them, even better!

God wants us to change medicine for *all* His children, young and old, from every nation throughout the earth. That's powerful! Let's join together on this mission and effortlessly bring the *hope* of healing to your patients — upgrading to a Heavenly White Coat!

It's time to move from wishful thinking to confident expectation that complete healing can flow through you to your patients as you stand in the gap and act as the Medical Intercessor God desires you to become. It's time to go be the light of the world and bring hope back into the darkness that has hijacked the medical system.

It's time to go forth and heal!

OUT OF ALIGNMENT

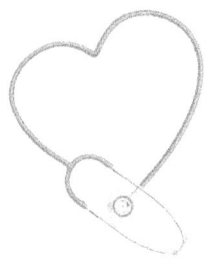

Chapter 1

BELIEVE IT OR NOT GOD IS PURSUING YOU

Come to Me, all you who labor and
are heavy laden, and I will give you rest.

— MATTHEW 11:28 (NKJV)

I was exhausted. For nearly two decades, I poured myself into the work I loved — medicine and caring for patients — until the strain of balancing my work and my personal life began taking a toll on my health that I couldn't ignore. Something had to give. Stepping away from my clinic and joining my husband in his business felt like the right decision at the time, but as the years passed, the absence of the calling I loved created a disconnect inside me. The weight of lost purpose grew heavier each day. I was drained, discouraged, and barely making it through one day at a time. My prayer became a constant whisper: *"Lord, what is my purpose now?"*

Then, in February 2024, everything shifted. I had an encounter with God that awakened something I thought I had lost forever.

For the first time in years, I felt free. I was present, energized, and suddenly aware that the passion for medicine I had buried was still alive. The joy that rose in me felt nothing short of miraculous.

What I didn't understand then was that this moment was only the beginning. God was preparing me for a story that He Himself would unfold — a journey where exhaustion would give way to miracles, and where the healer would become the healed. My encounter didn't just refresh me; it brought me into a deeper awareness of God's wisdom, peace, and power than anything I had known in my clinical training. Nothing in my medical training had prepared me for what He would show me in the months ahead.

In the year that followed, God pursued me with clarity and purpose. He realigned my heart, restored my identity, and began sending me into conversations and situations that revealed His assignment for me. He knew exactly what was missing in my life. He knew the purpose He had for me required stepping back into medicine — not in the same way as before, but with a renewed understanding of how He moves in the lives of His children. And He gave me an unmistakable call: pursue others who have drifted from their purpose, just as I had. Help them realign with Him, so He could restore their joy. When you've carried exhaustion for years, you learn to recognize it in others instantly. I didn't know it at the time, but one evening God would reflect my own story back to me through someone else's eyes — and that moment would confirm everything He had been preparing me to do.

It happened on a warm fall night in the backyard of my sister-in-law's home. Our children were running through the yard, laughing freely in the way only kids can. Their joy filled the air as I talked with Samantha, my sister-in-law's close friend.

She had a gentle, welcoming presence — the kind that immediately puts you at ease. But beneath her kindness, I noticed a quiet tiredness. A subtle strain around her eyes. A smile that carried more weight than she let on. It wasn't dramatic, but it was real. And I recognized it, because I had lived it. As we talked, she mentioned she was a doctor. Inside, I paused. All year long, God had been placing physicians in my path — not in hospitals or conferences, but in unexpected places where medicine wasn't even the topic. It had happened too many times to dismiss. And now here I was again, meeting another doctor for the first time in a place that felt completely ordinary, yet undeniably orchestrated. God's timing was too precise to ignore.

"What specialty are you in? Where do you work?" I asked.

She told me she was a family physician with a large corporate hospital system. As she described her role, I could hear the familiar tension between her calling and her current reality — a dissonance many of us have felt when the work that once gave life begins to drain it instead.

Sensing God's nudge, I gently asked, "When did you first feel called into healthcare?"

She paused, then began sharing her story — a story filled with passion, purpose, and the slow erosion of joy that often goes unnoticed until it's nearly gone.

And in that moment, I understood exactly why God brought us together that night.

This wasn't a coincidence. This was a calling for her, for me … and now for you.

A HEART-FOCUSED PHYSICIAN

"I knew when I was four that it was what I would do," Samantha told me, sipping her glass of iced tea as she reminisced. "My mother asked me several times as I grew up, 'What do you want to be? A princess? A model? Or a doctor?' It was our little joke.

And I would always bounce and twirl around and say, 'Doctor! Mommy, I want to be a doctor!'"

Samantha grew up on a farm far from town. "If we had minor or semi-major medical needs, my father would get creative with home remedies," she told me. "When I got a cut on my hand, he pulled out the super glue." We laughed at this.

"He always came up with some simple remedy to take care of his family with such love and gentleness, and that was inspiring." She went on to explain that she wanted to continue spreading that simple joy, taking care of others as a fully trained physician.

"But it's not so easy, is it?" she asked, shaking her head, her eyes now losing some of their humor.

"Why not?" I asked, curious. I had encountered plenty of my own frustrations as a medical provider, but I wondered what she would say.

She told me about a frustrating patient situation that represented a common obstacle many of us have encountered. A 10-year-old male patient had come into her clinic, and the boy's mother explained all the symptoms she'd noticed her son was experiencing. Dr. Samantha then asked the child if he could describe what he was experiencing — while working as quickly as possible. Under pressure, she knew she only had 19 minutes with each patient to assess, evaluate, diagnose, and recommend treatment — including the required paperwork.

"With that limited amount of time, you only get to gather a partial history. It's kind of like speed-dating," she remarked. We laughed at this description, though it was also an unfortunate truth.

However, there was an even greater problem. "Based on the conversations with the mother and the boy about the symptoms they described, I had a gut feeling that this little boy had asthma," she said. "When I have a feeling like that, I know it comes from God. I wanted to order a particular imaging and medical test to confirm my suspicion and get him on the right treatment."

However, we both knew that regardless of what would benefit the patient, the system doesn't support guidance by intuition. "Everything is a code," she said. "But there's not a 'gut feeling' code I can use when I'm charting. Unfortunately, I was out of time to find the exact billing code to ensure insurance approval of the imaging test I wanted to order for him. I don't know how many minutes I wasted scrolling through the endless list of ICD-10 codes and then attempting to locate the corresponding CPT codes to ensure I got insurance to approve my treatment plan."

The clock was ticking, and Dr. Samantha had to provide something for this mother and her son that could be approved. "I had to choose the third-best option for a treatment plan," she said, her voice tight with dismay. "That was our best chance at getting insurance approval. It's so frustrating because the treatment I was forced to give the patient will only help him feel slightly better. So, what do you think will happen? They'll have to come back, or they'll just accept the outcome as the best the child can feel, which is even worse. I hope they do come back." She sighed.

Samantha told me that if they did come back, she could get insurance to approve the next best option. But even then, they would have to come back another time before she could play the insurance-approval-process game to finally get them the best treatment — the one she knew they needed now!

"Ugh," I said, my heart filling with sympathy for both her and the family in this predicament. "That's heart-wrenching. It must feel so frustrating and discouraging."

"Yes," she said. "I often wish I had been born 50 or more years ago so I could treat patients as I'd like to. I'd have more than 19 minutes with them. I could make house calls and give them simple remedies. And the worst part is that even though our field has gained so much medical knowledge over the past 50 years, we are more restricted than ever in how we can apply it."

As we talked, I learned that Dr. Samantha had another struggle: Balancing her personal well-being with her career. I assumed this was one of the reasons she looked so tired. After she practiced medicine for a few years, she had become a mother. As she tried to balance raising little ones with a demanding profession, she became continually burned out.

"I felt a tug on my heart to live a more balanced life. I needed to prioritize caring for my own health and parenting my daughters," she said. "And of course, I wanted to continue being a physician."

In her eyes, she had three options. Option one was to stop working as a physician and focus solely on her family. However, the amount of student loan debt from attending medical school made that choice impossible.

Option two was to decrease her patient load and increase her time from 19 minutes per patient to 30 minutes per patient. She'd also need to cut back on some clinic hours. Unfortunately, physicians in her position were paid per patient, so this option would halve her salary. As with most of the American healthcare system, her employer valued profits over patient outcomes.

The third option was to open her own clinic, learn how to do business, find her own patients, and ultimately work many more hours building a business for a few years. However, while this might solve the length of time with the patient problem, it sure wouldn't give her the desired time with her precious children. And she realized building a successful business could take years and might not solve all her other concerns. Samantha knew some physicians who'd left corporate medicine and succeeded in starting their own small practices, yet she also knew others who became more miserable as the time they spent navigating business, payroll, legal boundaries, etc., pulled them away from their passion of providing quality patient care.

Ultimately, Samantha chose the second option. She gained a little more time with her patients, but at the cost of drastic financial change in her family's income.

You probably know it's a myth that physicians are taking in tons of money from their patients. The insurance takes the first cut, the corporation takes the next cut, liability insurance always gets a large chunk, and by the time the physician gets paid, there is not much left. It's a tough choice to make when you've paid nearly half a million dollars for your education, you're in your mid-30s, and your monthly student loan payments are more than your home mortgage. Factoring in the investment of their schooling, the cost of liability insurance, and the cost to maintain their licenses, our physicians earn far less than many other professions, despite the outrageous costs of medical care.

Samantha seemed resigned to her decision and determined to stay positive despite the difficult circumstances it put her in. As she spoke, I could hear her frustration but also her hope and determination. She was a fighter, and she wouldn't give up easily. She would find a way to make it all work.

SIMILAR STORIES INTERSECT

I could relate to Dr. Samantha's experience. When I worked for a physical therapist many years ago, I very quickly learned about the ugliness of insurance restrictions and the conflict they create between what we've been taught and what we set out to do as medical professionals.

I was only a few years into my professional career as a Certified Athletic Trainer when I had my first desire-versus-reality moment.

My career was fueled by a passion for the knee, prevention of knee injuries, and establishing full and complete recovery in athletes following ACL surgeries. This topic was near and dear to me since I'd experienced five knee surgeries in five years, three of which were ACL tears that occurred while playing basketball, my favorite sport.

Knees were, therefore, my favorite joint in the body, and I invested much of my time in school researching them. My master's thesis was focused on hip position and its effect on the alignment of the knee joint with regard to ACL injuries in female athletes, so I knew quite a bit about them. I loved to provide simple and effective therapy solutions for injured knees.

One day, the physical therapist I worked for was struggling to get his patient the outcomes she wanted, and she was continually experiencing knee pain throughout weeks of physical therapy. Knowing the knee was my passion, he asked me to take a look and determine why the patient could not overcome her pain.

Within a few minutes of assessment, it was very clear to me that she had a pelvic positioning issue that appeared to be caused by her right hip and lower back.

I eagerly told him about three simple steps the patient could implement to overcome her pain. This was exactly what I'd spent two years writing my master's thesis about, and it was the number-one method I'd used to overcome my own long journey of knee injuries.

To my dismay, he replied, "We cannot do any manual therapy to her low back or hips when she's here. She's been diagnosed with knee pain, not hip pain." He briefly educated me that insurance would deny any work we did on anything other than her knee and would not pay us for her therapy if we chose the treatment I'd recommended. She would have to go back to her doctor and see if he could change the diagnosis to "low back or hip pain" first.

"Unfortunately, that won't happen because the pain is in her knee, and she doesn't report any hip or back pain," he said.

In complete shock and disappointment, I realized that this patient would have to continue living in some pain when I knew without any doubt that we could get her out of pain within the next 20 minutes. Out of respect for the therapist, I only worked on the patient's knee and tried to think outside of the box as best as I could without violating any insurance orders. The patient improved, but I knew she would be back for continued therapy over the years because we had addressed only the current symptoms of her knee pain, not the cause.

From that day on, I knew I was not meant to work on patients who use marketplace health insurance as their payor. Too many limitations prevented these patients from getting proper care. Though it's been almost 20 years, I can still clearly remember the smell of that newly opened clinic, what the patient looked like, the clinic layout, where I was standing when I learned the truth about practicing medicine, and the jaw-dropping words that came out of my boss's mouth when he shared the reality of our situation.

I was shocked that an insurance company would have the upper hand over the trained medical provider who'd studied the body throughout years and years of schooling. Insurance competency was not part of my seven years of college because the profession of a Certified Athletic Trainer was unique. The traditional settings for athletic trainers paid us to evaluate, assess, treat, and set up injury prevention protocols by funds separate from insurance. To this day, my heart breaks for those providers who have to navigate insurance obstacles every day.

I also relate to Dr. Samantha in juggling the beautiful role of motherhood with the love for medicine and healing. I had attempted to provide excellent patient care by opening an independent cash-pay business while also trying to be a devoted mother for my three little children. The stress of doing both devastated my health. In 2016, I became so ill that I had to abruptly close my business that I loved so much. I had solved one problem yet created another.

God doesn't want us to solve one problem for Him at the cost of something else equally important. He wants us to prosper in all we do. He wants to show His Glory through us in all aspects of our life — work, health, and family. This is exactly the reason God called me back into medicine and to write this book: to offer a better solution for balancing all that God calls us to.

Over the past year, God has been delivering me visions, dreams, and plans to share with you. Keep reading, and you will encounter the love letter He has for you. He loves you! **He chose you to care for His children and wants to take back the health of the human body by healing the heart and mind of the medical provider.** He wants to heal the heart of His beloved child inside of that white coat!

A SIMPLE SOLUTION

The solution is simple — Partnership. You are created on purpose for a purpose, and the desire to heal and work in medicine is your unique spiritual gifting that God planted in you. **And you were never meant to operate alone.**

I believe that if we bring medicine back to God's original design, relying on the guidance and partnership from above and combining it with the extensive knowledge and skills we have gained, we can provide amazing medical care, no matter the obstacles -- all while living a life filled with balance and abundant joy.

The Lord wants to work *with* you in partnership. In Mark 16:19 (NKJV), God worked with the early Christians and added His power to their efforts. We are called to be co-workers with God (1 Corinthians 3:9, NIV). The Greek root word used here is *synergeo*, which means to work with or work together. When you choose to co-labor and partner with God, you will navigate over the obstacles of today's medical system and fulfill your purpose in the role of healing as the Creator originally intended. There is no greater partner to co-labor with than the omniscient, all-knowing One!

Throughout this book, I will show you how simple it is to 100x your healing impact with just one change — intentional, interactive, *synergeo*. It will blow your mind to discover how simple and effective this solution is. Your work doesn't have to be so hard. In fact, you will soon learn that working in alignment with His purpose for you is incredibly simple.

It's important to note that learning to partner with God isn't just about helping you strengthen your practice. It is about bringing *you* back to your true God-given purpose, which releases countless spiritual blessings.

With His partnership, the patient solutions also become simple. The burden of finding more effective patient solutions and strategies is removed when you work *with Him*. You will renew your strength, soar on wings like eagles, and run and not grow weary (Isaiah 40:31, NKJV).

White Coat Revival is designed to help you identify how and why you got into a place of misalignment with God in your profession, show you how to pivot to provide the care you desire to deliver, and give you some steps to become a co-laborer in healing with the Creator of the human body Himself.

DUALITY OF DESIRES

As a healer, you likely operate from two desires. On one hand, you strive to gain extraordinary knowledge and skills to be the best you can be to heal those in need, all while navigating your professional guidelines, rules, and regulations (embedded in your mind). On the other hand, you desire more evidence of God's presence and promises in your life as you dedicate yourself to serving Him through your love for medicine (embedded in your heart). This duality creates a chasm between your mind and your heart, which also leads to a perceived separation between science and Spirit.

The good news is that God knows this duality exists in your life and has designed His amazingly simple partnership solution to resolve it — helping you soar over your professional obstacles without striving. **His design includes *both* science (gaining knowledge) and Spirit (partnership with Him).**

This starts not with trying to change the industry, but with changing the most important part of the industry — *you*. Most importantly, healing your heart and your mind.

Changing medicine starts from the inside out by realigning *you* with God. Only then can you start experiencing the gifts that come with this alignment, including hope, balance, joy, fulfillment, and best of all, peace.

> *Changing medicine starts from the inside out by realigning you with God.*

With that in mind, I've also provided an example of what alignment looks like in practice so you can begin imagining how you can use your partnership with the Great Physician in your own day-to-day work. We'll look at the philosophy behind how this partnership works, and then you'll get an overview of the 7 Alignments as a transformational process for aligning with God. This chapter prepares you to move on to the next section, in which you'll work through each of the 7 Alignments, one by one, to create your foundation as a Medical Intercessor who stands in the gap between God and your patient. You'll realign with the Great Physician in a way that will give you 100x healing impact and reignite your God-given purpose to heal according to His plan.

THE 7 ALIGNMENTS: AN OVERVIEW

These Alignments are a series of steps that build on each other to fully align you with God's will and the purpose He placed in you for His promise to be fulfilled here on earth as in heaven. They were created to eliminate the complexities that have arisen due to various misalignments and to restore you to His simple design. By following each step, you can become 100 percent aligned with God as His partner. It's important that you proceed in order because each step teaches you things you will build upon in the next.

The 7 Alignments are as follows:

1. **Align with God's vision.** Aligning with God's will for your life, your unique calling into medicine, and His vision for you to be the vessel of healing, will empower you through His partnership according to God's plan.

2. **Align with the purpose God intended for you.** Reconnect with your original heart's desire and your God-given purpose as an essential ingredient in God's vision. Remember: He specifically designed you as a promise for His will to be done here on earth through you. When you are aligned with your purpose (which is also part of His purpose), your energy, your joy, and your peace are restored.

3. **Align your soul with your spirit.** Unite with God's Living Word, so your faith in His perfect design will sanctify your soul — your mind, will, emotions, and knowledge. This alignment enables you to be made new so you can operate from the mind of Christ, just as Jesus demonstrated when He was in the world.

4. **Align your expectation with the God of all hope.** Redefine the hope you offer your patient from wishful thinking to a confident expectation for complete

healing — freeing them from their disease, illness, injury, or infirmity. This hope is how you integrate faith into medicine.

5. **Align with God's love and stand in the gap.** Pair your healing authority with God's abundant love and surrender yourself fully as a conduit to flow His love and His will for complete healing to your patient. Love moves mountains — challenges in the exam room fade away.

6. **Align your mind with your heart.** Recommit to leading with your heart's desire (who God made you to be) instead of leading with your mind (misguided knowledge). Recode your mind to remove the limitations from which you have been operating and leading, and instead, lead with your heart and God's vision.

7. **Align science with Spirit and partner with heaven.** Reconnecting the heart of medicine to the heart of God fuses Spirit with science, empowering you to heal beyond your own strength. You will walk in your purpose and your power, exercise the authority God has given you as a Medical Intercessor, and intercede in healing every patient by balancing your extraordinary knowledge with God's omniscient wisdom.

Are you excited to get started? I know I am! Let's dive in!

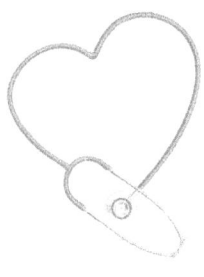

Chapter 2

IT'S OKAY TO WANT MORE

The Lord is my shepherd; I shall not want. He makes me to lie down in green pastures; He leads me beside the still waters. He restores my soul; He leads me in the path of righteousness For His name's sake.

— PSALM 23:1-3 (NKJV)

Before we get into the 7 Alignments, it is important to address any lies that may have come into your mind over the years. Too often, we journey through life operating from a wrong belief or a lie that God never intended for us to hold onto. In Chapter 4, I will unpack the lie that led me to close the doors of my clinic and leave my passion, medicine. I operated from a wrong belief that I created in my own mind — about a Biblical principle that I mis-understood — and made a decision that took me off track from my purpose. I want to share it with you in hopes that you will see what similar lies could be holding you back, too. This awareness will make your transformation process go more smoothly.

Let's look at the well-known Bible passage: Psalm 23. It starts with, "The Lord is my shepherd; I shall not want."

"I shall not want" is preceded by "The Lord is my shepherd." Therefore, **when** the Lord is my shepherd, **then** I shall not want.

The word "shall" is not a decision you can make or a decision you can choose. It's a gift God gives you. You are given the gift of not wanting **when** you trust Him and partner with Him every moment of every day.

I think many of us can very quickly answer, "Yes, the Lord is my shepherd." But this answer can be one of acknowledgement alone. A shepherd leads its sheep by the power of an established relationship. Jesus addressed His Father often in the Gospels. He talked about God as His Father, indicating He was in a relationship with Him to make decisions about what He is to do and what He is not to do.

The Lord is your shepherd **when** you are in a relationship with Him — when you are in partnership and co-laboring with Him — not just acknowledging His existence and reaching to Him once in a great while, but instead in consistent *synergeo*.

Let's think about this: I know I am writing this book because we all want solutions in healthcare. I know you want change. You want better patient outcomes. You want more respect. You want more life balance. You want more God in your workplace.

What do you do, then, if you are wanting? Does this type of wanting even apply to that verse?

After all, you are not wanting earthly things; you are just wanting better solutions to heal your patients. That's why God placed you in medicine — to serve your patients by seeking more knowledge to produce better outcomes. I agree that this type of wanting is not a selfish desire; it's a sacrifice. I am here to tell you the *wanting* is exactly what God is calling your attention to. That wanting is a heavenly knock. Not something to rationalize away.

The reason we are wanting change is that we are not embracing the Lord completely as our shepherd. His leadership requires partnership or *synergeo* that I discussed in Chapter 1. When we are not partnering or co-laboring with Him, we are left wanting more because that's how He designed us — to be in partnership with Him.

You probably feel that you have done an excellent job seeking knowledge, skills, and expertise to be positioned as the hands and feet for God to bring healing here on earth. You have answered His call by positioning yourself in healthcare and are committed to being the best healer you can be. And you may even believe your obedience to this is the answer from God to your patient for healing. After all, this is your purpose.

We need to remove the lie that you have to strive to find solutions *on your own* to better serve your patient — that God gave you the gifts and talents to gain the expertise needed to heal your patient, and that's all there is. God has so much more for you! He never intended for you to do it alone.

The wanting more that you feel is because something is still missing. God does want you to have more — Him! He wants you to *partner with Him*! He wants to co-labor with you every day, with every patient.

You remain wanting until you form an interactive, co-working relationship with Him. When this ongoing relationship is established, just like a sheep follows its shepherd, then you will know the Lord is your shepherd, and *you shall not want* — and you will have the *gift* of not wanting. It is a place of contentment, a fulfillment of peace like no other.

THE PARTNER WHO CHANGES EVERYTHING

Your obedience to a vocation in medicine and your storehouse filled with extraordinary knowledge needed to care for your patients **are only half of the equation**.

God's partnership is the other half of the equation. The wanting that you experience happens because you lack the second part of the equation. 1 part + 1 part does not equal 2. God's math is multiplication. It equals 100x healing impact!

Phenomenal patient outcomes and your life filled with contentment and peace come only through co-laboring with Him.

When you let Him partner with you and take the lead, you can work "*from Him, through Him, and for Him*" (Romans 11:36, NKJV). That's when His Glory is displayed. God wants to show off through you! He wants you to be positioned to show His Glory! He doesn't want you to carry the weight of responsibility for your patients' healing all on your own. That was never His plan.

God wants to show off through you

God told me, "Marilyn, I blessed you with that [medical] knowledge, so you would partner with Me." Ever since I responded to that invitation to partner with Him, I have seen countless healing miracles, been filled with an inner joy that overflows, and experienced a peace and stillness I had not known prior to that day. The switch I made from thinking I had to strive to gain more knowledge to ensure I healed my patient to realizing I just needed to partner with the Great Physician exponentially increased my healing impact! I have witnessed miracle after miracle.

You can too!

He has blessed you with knowledge of His prize creation — the human body — and His partnership is the key to knowing the exact solution for each patient's problem, overcoming the obstacles within the medical system, and restoring your joy. You

His partnership is the key to knowing the exact solution for each patient's problem, overcoming the obstacles within the medical system, and restoring your joy.

don't need to strive in wanting anymore. You don't have to take a pay cut, change your job, open a business, or leave medicine to seek that freedom. God has you right where He wants you.

I know. My entire life has changed. I was a very dedicated student of the body. I spent countless days filling my storehouse of knowledge, purchasing the next best modality, getting certified in the newest approach, breaking the chains of insurance obstacles, and opening a business to ensure I did everything I could to heal my patients and free them from the chains of injury. However, that only led me to eventually close my dream clinic, leaving me in no position to heal any patient.

You don't have to make difficult, heartbreaking decisions like Dr. Samantha or I did, but you do have to answer that knock. That knocking is because there is more for you — a partner waiting to join you!

Answering that knock will bring you power, authority, and compassion like the medical world has never seen before.

A PAUSE TO PREPARE FOR ALIGNMENT

At the end of every Alignment chapter, I have included an Alignment Pause. This pause is for you to stop and reflect, then take action to redirect. Some of the pauses will ask you to ask God specific questions; others will encourage you to dig deep within your own heart. It is important for you to locate a quiet place and create intentional time. Some of the pauses will take you a minute or two, and some will take much longer. I know God will redeem your time tenfold, so please trust this process and enjoy the transformation ahead.

If your mind is swirling with the thought so that you are unable to hear God's "still, small voice" (1 Kings 19:12, NKJV), it is important to start with a few minutes of just focusing on your breathing, not on your thoughts. This helps prepare your mind to receive from God.

Before we get into the Alignment Pause, I want to introduce you to something fascinating that God engineered into the body. He designed us to hear His voice and embedded an important "switch" within our nervous system to do so — the vagus nerve. In the simplest terms, the vagus nerve is like a switch within our body to move from striving — the sympathetic nervous system response for "fight or flight" — to a stillness posture — a parasympathetic system response for "rest and digest." The lifestyle so many of us operate in these days is fight or flight, day in and day out, but in order to hear God's still, small voice, we must be in a parasympathetic nervous system state.

There are many simple techniques to shift into a parasympathetic state. Be sure to download the supplemental content for this book. In that download, I include a great resource for some of these techniques.

The simple technique we will use right now is focusing on our breath. When we shift our mind from our thoughts to focusing only on breathing, we will feel our breath go in and out, and we will begin to make that shift to a parasympathetic state.

Let's do our first alignment pause together. Before we begin, grab a pen and a notebook to write down any important messages or insights you receive.

To begin, just start feeling your breath go in through your nose and out through your mouth. Then start to breathe out longer than you breathe in — four seconds of breath in, seven seconds of breath out, four seconds of breath in, seven seconds of breath out. Repeat that a few more times.

Now, we are going to ask God a question. We're going to ask God if there are any lies about yourself that you are operating from that are hindering your relationship with Him.

So, say, "Lord, are there any lies that I am believing about myself that are hindering our relationship?"

Sit in stillness with Him. Write down any images, even faint ones, that come to mind, anything new that comes into your mind. Take note of anything you feel, sense, see, or hear. Write it down without editing. It's important to not edit.

When God partners with you, you will be amazed how something new comes into your thinking that you have not thought about before. Sometimes, it will be so simple that you may not think it's from God. Sometimes, He will show you something that you never once thought about, but you will know in your spirit that it's spot on.

When we remove a lie, it leaves a void within that we need to fill, so it's very important to now ask God, "What do You want to show me that is true about me that will create a stronger relationship with You?"

Same thing as above: Write down any images that come to mind, anything new that comes into your mind. Take note of anything you feel, sense, see, or hear. Write it down without editing.

Hopefully, you now have learned something new about yourself: a lie and a truth. It's important to now activate the truth. Let's put that truth in place of the lie and recode your mind. Simply, say out loud, *"I release the lie (insert the lie you wrote down), and I receive the truth (insert the truth you wrote down)."*

By removing the lies, you create new neuro pathways in your brain that change your thinking so that you can align with God's full promises for you. This is what the Apostle Paul instructs us to do in Romans 12:2 (NKJV): "... Be transformed by the renewing of your mind, that you may prove what is that good and acceptable and perfect will of God."

Neuroscience researchers have recognized the power of brain training. This technique of asking God for the wisdom to recode your brain is how science explains the power of renewing your mind mentioned in scripture. I recommend you read Dr. Caroline Leaf's book *Switch on Your Brain*[1], which will help you understand why this technique works and why I have Alignment Pauses at the end of each chapter as an essential tool to transform your stressful days into joyful days!

Let your alignment transformation begin as you develop a beautiful relationship with your Shepherd.

RESTORING ALIGNMENT WITH GOD: THE 7 ALIGNMENTS™

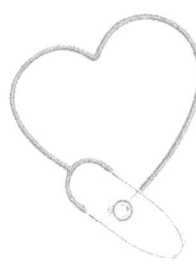

Chapter 3

ALIGNMENT 1: ALIGN WITH GOD'S VISION

"For My thoughts are not your thoughts, Nor are your ways My ways,"
says the LORD. "For as the heavens are higher than the earth, so are
My ways higher than your ways, And My thoughts than your thoughts."

— ISAIAH 55:8–9 (NKJV)

Instead of longing to do more for your patients, imagine living each day knowing that whatever you need, you will receive. You don't need to scramble around for answers. You don't need to worry about legalities or restrictions. Your day will go smoothly, and you'll go home each day feeling fulfilled, knowing you made a wonderful difference in the lives of those who needed you. You'll be at peace, understanding that you're working in a role that not only was made for you — you were made for it! You have every skill you need, and when you encounter something outside your area of skill or expertise, all you have to do is consult your partner, an expert who wants to help you.

That sounds wonderful, doesn't it? How can you get a situation like that?

This first Alignment is the first step toward achieving that reality.

God's vision is to work through you. You are created in His image. He gave you gifts, talents, and many abilities. He gave you the Holy Spirit as a powerful guide to lead you exactly where He wants you.

Knowing this, every day, we should be asking, "Lord, where do you want to use me today? How can I reflect your love today?" Last chapter, I discussed God as a partner. In this chapter, I want you to think of Him as the best CEO ever to work for. He is clear on His plans and every decision. He orchestrates everything to set you up for prosperity. He thinks of you as His Masterpiece. Follow His lead!

ARE YOU WHERE YOU WANT TO BE?

Let's think about the current health of your career compared to your original ideal — the vision you were so excited to pursue many years ago.

What was the original vision that gave you the strength and focus to make it through all the late nights and challenging coursework during your education?

You sure didn't dedicate many years of study and pay hundreds of thousands of dollars for your education, sacrifice your social life, skip nights of sleep, bury your head in textbooks, drink an insane amount of caffeine to ensure you studied enough to pass your licensure exam, and even postpone starting your family for nothing. You did it out of obedience to God's calling for you and God's promises for both heaven and here on earth.

I bet you envisioned yourself caring for people in one way or another, providing a solution to a problem, or healing or eradicating a disease, illness, or injury. Perhaps you related a little to Jesus healing the blind man or coming alongside the lame who couldn't walk, or maybe you simply thought that people who wanted healing would find you and you would be able to make their dreams come true and help them. Perhaps, like me, you were inspired by your childhood doctor who poured out their love for you and seemed to really listen to your pain and take it away.

My childhood doctor, Dr. Jim, was one of two local docs who served all of our small town, plus the neighboring towns. Dr. Jim was a sweet man. He always welcomed us with a warm and compassionate smile. His voice was one that spoke the language of peace, never fear. He was a patient man, not filled with busyness or worry about all the paper documentation that's seen so often in the physician's office nowadays. Dr. Jim was a great influence on my love for medicine because he radiated godly love as he served his patients.

I wanted to be just like him. I'm sure you wanted to be just like your own role models too.

And yet... how does where you are today compare with your big dreams of caring for your patients? Do you feel off track? Does it feel as if everything is out of your control? Most of us can relate to the struggle of feeling misalignment between our heart's desire and the reality of working in the healthcare system.

WHEN THE DREAM DOESN'T MATCH REALITY

If navigating through the healthcare maze seems way off track from the ideals you held when you started caring for others, you are not alone. In the process of writing this book, I connected with thousands of genuinely loving souls who felt off track from the dream they set out on. Unfortunately, simple and complete healing of the body is not the main focus in today's medical industry.

Through the stories shared by people like you, I became painfully aware of the complexity and challenges you navigate every day as you try to give your patients the best care possible and how often you feel like you're failing. Not only that, but you're starting to be disrespected and avoided by the same people you have dedicated your life to serving: your patients.

Patient trust in doctors declined substantially between 1966 and 2012 and even more so since the pandemic.[2] This unfortunate reality hit home when I saw a satirical cartoon of a physician sitting across from a patient, and the patient was saying to the physician, "Doctor, please just tell me the truth." The doctor in the cartoon responded, "Sorry, the medical board will take away my license if I do that. You'll just have to trust the lies I'm telling you or I can't see you anymore."

What's the point of having an amazing amount of knowledge, expertise, and experience if insurance; large, profit-focused corporations; pharmaceutical companies; and legal restrictions supersede all of that grand knowledge? And you are left positioned in front of your patient to say, "Here is a so-so diagnosis or treatment plan. I know it's not the best, and I don't even align with it, but sorry, you just have to accept it."

Chained in a Tug of War

Today, with the corporate side of medical care, big pharma, insurance, and governing boards that threaten to revoke licenses if we bring our faith into work, we fight an internal tug-of-war.

Our inner desire to care for the whole person pulls us in one direction, while the industry's limitations often force us to deliver rubbish, second-rate, substandard medical care, as Dr. Samantha's story in Chapter 1 depicts. **In these instances, we experience a double mindset or a disconnect between our heart's desire and our mind's training that keeps us from being our true, authentic self.**

This inauthenticity compels us to create different versions of ourselves depending upon the environment. As we veer off path from our God-given purpose, we risk living independently from our Father's plan for us. We present a different self at home than we do at work or in our community. We show up differently with our children. We show up differently in our church. These disparate versions of our identity need to stop. We are called to be the beautiful souls God created us to be, no matter what environment we journey through each day. As we accept these inauthentic fragments within ourselves, we also have to deal with the complexities of a medical industry that, as a whole, has also become misaligned and off track from its original purpose — to bring healing to those who need it.

What happens when we and our industry are misaligned with God's vision — for us and for medicine?

To show me this, God gave me a heart-wrenching vision: a person wearing a medical white coat, sitting on a chair and wrapped in a thick layer of fog. Attached to their wrists and ankles, pulling them down into a hunched position in the chair, were chains labeled "insurance," "liability," and "pharmaceuticals."

In the same fog, their patient stood in front of them seeking help. The white coat attempted to look up at their patient but could offer them nothing due to the chains holding them down. The patient's agony and frustration were plastered all over their face. It was a helpless situation.

FIGURE 3.1 A CHAINED AND HELPLESS WHITE COAT.

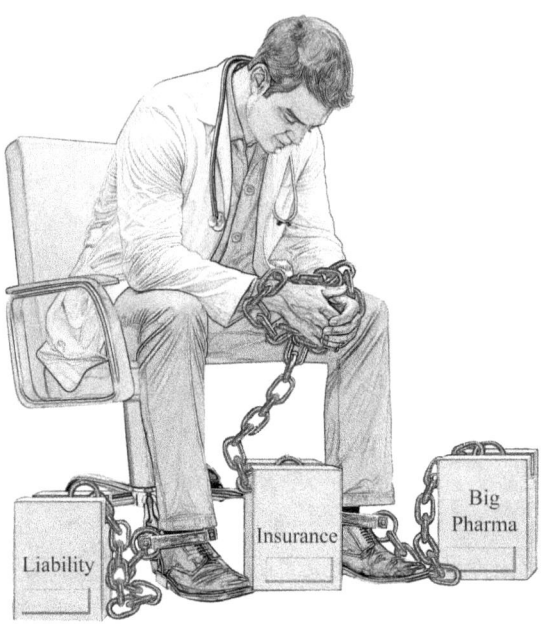

God has set you out on this purposeful professional path to care for His children, your patients. Unfortunately, when you are still wearing the chains in the current medical system, you end up presenting your patient with a solution sometimes wrapped in a lie or incomplete truth, and providing them with limited hope for their potential to be freed from the disease, injury, or illness that you assess. You unintentionally create fear and hopelessness more often than not when you simply abide by the rules, regulations, and greed that fill our medical system. This isn't where any of us want to be.

The great news is that God loves you and is pursuing you and drawing you in close to Him and reigniting your heart's desire to serve Him through your patients. He has been with you all along. I know God is pursuing you and looking to embrace you and bring you back into

> *God is pursuing you and looking to embrace you and bring you back into alignment with Him.*

alignment with Him. His ways are better! Throughout this book, you will discover His full vision and the simple strategies He has for you to transform medicine back to His original intent.

And He knows that to transform our industry back to what He intended, the first thing we need to know is how we got here.

HOW MEDICINE WENT OFF TRACK

In 2024, God shared with me two powerful visions to help me understand what has gone wrong in the medical industry.

The Two Pedestals: An Individual's Path to Truth

In one of the visions God showed me, I saw two pedestals standing in the middle of two parallel pathways. On each pedestal was a leader.

FIGURE 3.2 PEDESTAL VISION

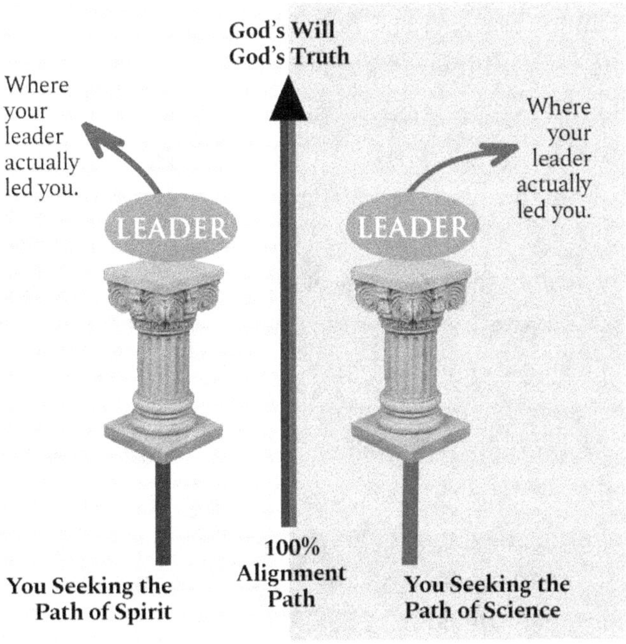

God's Will
God's Truth

Where your leader actually led you.

Where your leader actually led you.

LEADER

LEADER

100% Alignment Path

You Seeking the Path of Spirit

You Seeking the Path of Science

The two pedestals look similar, but they represent the two pathways we commonly take throughout our life journey. Each pedestal has a corresponding pathway for seeking the truth of that particular subject.

One pathway, the **Path of Spirit**, represents how we seek truth about God. We, or in some cases, our parents, chose a leader to guide us along that pathway via church (i.e., a minister or a religion).

The other pathway, the **Path of Science**, symbolized how we set out on our journey seeking the knowledge to become the medical professional we desired to be, with hopes of learning how to become equipped to heal or cure. We chose a profession, college, specialty, and approach to medicine. Therefore, we chose a leader or system to trust and follow and started our journey without looking back.

In my vision, God showed me a person standing before the two pedestals. God explained that when we set out on a path to seek truth, it is our nature to first choose a leader to guide us. The leader, standing on the pedestal (representative of expertise), would teach us, and hopefully lead us to know truth.

The vision illustrates the real problem: We've been led to believe that the Path of Spirit and the Path of Science are two different journeys. As a result, we chose one type of leader for one area of expertise and another type of leader

> *We've been led to believe that the Path of Spirit and the Path of Science are two different journeys.*

for the other area of expertise. We believed the spiritual leader would teach us spiritual truths and trusted that they were an authority in their field and would help us understand God better. And we believed the same thing about the medical leader. We believed they, too, as an authority in their field, would lead us to the truth about how to care for the human body and how God designed the body to heal.

Unfortunately, by following one leader for one thing and another leader for the other, we didn't realize that the truth lies in the middle of the Path of Spirit and the Path of Science. It encompasses *both* things at once. God is not divided, and neither is truth. Neither human authority in these pathways knows the entire truth, yet we expect them to. Without realizing it, we divided our focus and created a chasm between our faith and our profession, separating the Path of Spirit from the Path of Science.

Instead of following two separate paths at once, we should be following a single path. When we are focused on God alone, He will guide us *to and from* leaders throughout our journey of seeking truth, spiritually and vocationally.

The Overswung Pendulum: An Ages-Long Evolution

The previous vision of the pedestals shows the journey we've taken from an individual perspective. Now, let's look at our industry as a whole. God showed me a second vision that illustrated the evolution of the medical field through the ages.

The discipline of medicine swings back and forth like a big pendulum between spirit and science.

There are two recognized approaches to healthcare that mirror the two principles characterizing the two pedestals: spirit and science. The discipline of medicine swings back and forth like a big pendulum between spirit and science. Sometimes, spirit is the overswung side, and science is ignored or downplayed. Other times, science is the overswung side, and spirit is ignored or downplayed.

What often happens is that when people recognize the flaws in an approach, they overcorrect and go too far to the other side of the spectrum. As a result, they move from one extreme to another, and neither is correct.

FIGURE 3.3 THE OVERSWUNG PENDULUM: APPROACHES TO MEDICINE

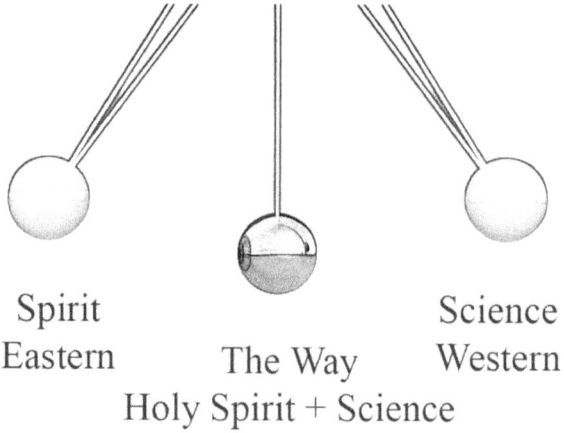

Spirit   Science

Eastern   The Way   Western

Holy Spirit + Science

To understand the overswung pendulum, I embarked on a research journey to learn where these two common approaches to medicine originated and identify the influences causing the pendulum to become overswung.

Many biblical scholars say man has existed for approximately 6,000 years, and for the sake of the timeline in this book, we'll agree. When I started digging into the research available to me online, I learned it wasn't until 700 BC, almost 4,000 years after the beginning of civilization, that the Greek civilization emerged with a focus on rational thinking and reasoning as an approach to medicine. They thirsted for logic-based decisions, and their curiosity paved the way for many math and science disciplines that are still foundational today.

Ancient records show that the Greeks established early medical schools and recognized medicine as an independent discipline. Alcmaeon, a Greek philosopher who lived around 500 BC, proposed that illness might be a result of environmental problems, nutrition, or lifestyle, despite what had been believed for the previous 4,000 years, which focused solely on repelling evil spirits as the most popular approach to medicine and answer to healing.

The two motivations that encouraged the ancient Greeks to seek healing and promote it separately from repelling evil spirits were war and the Olympic Games. Due to the observation of injuries from these events, they recognized a pattern of injury and illness that were not related to evil spirits but instead resulted from more observable causes, such as force. In this era, the Greeks focused on both physical and mental well-being.[3]

During the 4,000 years prior to Greek science and reasoning, medicine and healing were largely a cultural and spiritual reliance on divine intervention to ward off evil spirits, as well as some cultural recipes with herbs and balms. Therefore, I would best estimate that the start of what we call Western medicine has been swinging, to use the pendulum analogy, for just over 2,000 years.

Meanwhile, many cultures did not follow the lead of the Greeks and continued to evolve what we more commonly known as Eastern medicine or ancient medicine. These cultures created their own beliefs based on cultural habits and teachings and advanced to much more than just warding off evil spirits. Those cultures instead developed what they believed to be natural and whole-body care that included a spirit, mind or soul, and body healing approach. Unfortunately, most Eastern cultures' healing practices involve counterfeit spirits or other practices that do not align with the one true God. When God showed me that the Eastern side of the pendulum was overswung, he was referencing the increase in spiritual practices that do not align with Him and His Holy Spirit, in the name of Jesus. The God of the Trinity is the only source of pure miraculous healing.

Patients are seeking healing, and the current obstacles in Western medicine, leading to very poor patient outcomes, have prompted patients and practitioners to seek alternative therapies at a very high rate. Unfortunately, the presence of God's Holy Spirit in alternative therapies has been minimal, and many counterfeit spirits have been invited into this approach to healing. This spiritual side, too, has led to an overswung pendulum away from God's balanced approach.

Neither of these overswung solutions is the approach God desires. One side without the other simply creates more problems and does not fully resolve the true problem. Instead, God desires a balanced pendulum that includes both the blessing of your science-based knowledge and the power of the Holy Spirit.

RELEASE YOURSELF FROM DECEPTION

God's vision for healthcare and healing is very different from man's vision that is currently ruling the medical system as we know it today. The truth is that when you partner with Him and take on the mind of Christ in the presence of your patients, God's love, compassion, and hope for healing can be expressed and activated in a much bigger way.

> *When you partner with Him and take on the mind of Christ in the presence of your patients, God's love, compassion, and hope for healing can be expressed and activated in a much bigger way.*

Recognize the Misleading

Unfortunately, our leaders, no matter how good their intent, live in the same fallen world we live in, and they are not perfect. As a result, even with the best of intentions, they see only their part of the equation and may be unaware that there is another half of the equation as well. They can become misguided, in turn misguiding us. Whether or not they are misguided, we might continue believing they and their fragmented worldview are all we can rely on, without realizing that doing so may lead us away from truth.

Many scriptures warn against blindly trusting a human leader. Here are just three of them:

1. "It is better to trust in the Lord than to put confidence in man" (Psalm 118:8, NKJV).
2. "And my speech and my preaching *were* not with persuasive words of human wisdom, but in demonstration of the Spirit and of power, that your faith should not be in the wisdom of men but in the power of God" (1 Corinthians 2:4–5, NKJV).
3. "The fear of man brings a snare, but whoever trusts in the LORD shall be safe" (Proverbs 29:25 NKJV).

This is how our journey through medicine ended up way out of alignment with God's will. We can't try to follow pathways created by man because, good intentions or not, they are incomplete. Instead, we need to follow God's will, which is the 100 percent alignment path that travels between the two man-made pedestals.

We need to recognize where we've accepted some information that just isn't true and how it's affecting all our decisions. Deception can happen in such small ways at first that it is nearly imperceptible. It can sometimes take a while to see what's happening. Now that we do see it, we need to get back on track with the truth, and we need to do it soon.

Ground Yourself in Truth

Knowing how we've been misled, we can start releasing ourselves from the false limits that deception has imposed on us.

We can pivot away from relying only on flawed human leaders and turn back to the truth, keeping our eyes on God and trusting His guidance.

The best compass you can reference is the truth found in scripture and with God, who dwells in you and walks with you. Other people might offer some guidance at

> *The best compass you can reference is the truth found in scripture and with God, who dwells in you and walks with you.*

times, but they are travelers on the same path, seeking the same truth you are. You can't take the risk of putting all your faith in a potentially misguided, misaligned human authority. If you rely too much on the human teacher and forget to use the compass that God gave you — the Living Word, His scripture — you can end up way off the path you intended to be on.

I invite you in this moment to stop in your tracks, pivot, and turn away from the misguided journey and back toward God. Draw near to Him. Just like we did in Chapter 2, you can release the lie, replace it with truth, and create new neural pathways in your brain that change your thinking.

This pivot point is a blessing from Him. It is the moment God has been waiting for. He is never here to shame you. He already knows the flaws of humanity. He knows you were misled, and He was making good out of evil more often than you realize. If you are reading this book right now, you are exactly where God wants you. You are listening to His call, and you are ready for a new lesson from Him. This is an amazing moment because He is pursuing you and pulling you back into alignment with Him.

The most important thing to remember is that the solution isn't all up to you or the human leaders you've been relying on. In fact, thinking it is all up to humans is part of the problem. The solution is actually much simpler, and to find it, all you need to do is let go of your fragmented, overcomplicated worldview and put your trust in someone who knows exactly what to do — the One who created everything.

WHO IS MORE IMPORTANT THAN *HOW*

It's funny how the seemingly small lessons we learn in life are often bigger than we realize. This was one of those times for me.

After my children were born, I took a seven-year hiatus from working in sports medicine to work with my husband in his businesses and have a better family balance while the kids were little.

During that time, I was exposed to my husband's favorite business strategy from a book he studied, called *Who Not How*, by Dan Sullivan.[4] Quoting part of that strategy, my husband would often say, "It is who, not how."

He explained to me that success comes as a result of *who* we partner with or hire, not *how* we come up with the solution ourselves. It's not all up to us. **If we try to make all of those decisions or figure it all out ourselves, coming up with the *how* would take forever.** In addition, when we work outside our expertise, our solutions are limited because our knowledge is limited. This influence from Dan Sullivan became one of our strongest business strategies, which resulted in great levels of success.

Success comes as a result of who we partner with or hire, not how we come up with the solution ourselves.

Implementing this strategy is much simpler when you work with someone who is already an expert and you approach business obstacles or growth goals together. So often, we assume that with our knowledge, we just need to start looking at how to solve the problems. And yet, what we really need to look at is whether or not we have the *right people* with the *right expertise and experience* at the table to solve the problems. It doesn't matter how much we know about our subject if the problem we're trying to solve is related to something completely different, or if we don't have the experience needed to solve it.

A Pivot Point for a Company

Here's a perfect illustration of this *who, not how* strategy at work in a real situation.

Everyone knows how successful Apple Inc. has been. We just assume that's always been the case, right? Yet I was surprised to learn that this super-successful business, which is featured in so many business cases as an example to follow, almost failed in the mid-1980s and 1990s.

During that period, Steve Jobs, the company's visionary founder, left Apple and started a new company called NeXT Inc. with hopes of making a new vision come true. In his absence, Apple floundered. Though its products were user-friendly, sleek, and used advanced technology, Apple struggled with underpowered hardware, stiff competition from IBM, tension among the co-owners and executives, problems with business partners, egos, and so on. Meanwhile, NeXT, like any fledgling business, was also struggling against market obstacles of its own.

Then Apple's CEO at the time, Gil Amelio, made a brilliant decision to purchase NeXT and bring Steve Jobs back, realigning Apple with the visionary who had founded it.

This decision enabled the company to pivot and regain its lost market position. Mr. Amelio understood that the *how* couldn't be fixed until the right *who* was at the helm.

Even knowing how successful this strategy was — not only for my husband and me but for a huge company like Apple — I had no idea it would also apply in the spiritual realm. And yet, recently, it occurred to me... why wouldn't it?

What if we've been thinking about this in a way that's just making it more complicated, when really, it's as simple as a single choice of *who*?

THE RIGHT LEADER WILL TRANSFORM MEDICINE

As Apple learned, the leader whose vision you choose to align with is the difference between clarity and confusion. Our situation is similar.

It's Meant to Be Simple

Now it's time to share one of the more fun spiritual encounters I had with God. In February 2024, I received a vision in which I was hanging out with Jesus up on a cloud, high above the earth. We were sitting on the edge of the cloud, like you would when you sit on the tailgate of a truck, swinging our legs off the edge. I had the same feeling I would experience on a beautiful summer evening after a hard day of work on my parents' farm unloading hay bales. The peace was the reward of a well-deserved rest.

On the cloud, I was sitting shoulder to shoulder with Jesus, and we were looking down at the earth. I saw people moving in erratic patterns. I understood that it was the movement of white coats and patients journeying through the current medical system in hopes of finding healing for diseases, illnesses, or ailments with great exhaustion and minimal solutions. It was so peaceful up on that cloud, but I could feel the stress in the motion of the people down on the earth.

Jesus said to me, "Marilyn, that down there is a rat race."

Then I glanced back down at the earth and saw two people in different parts of the world standing perfectly still with their arms up above their heads, elbows straight and hands pressed together, standing in complete balance and stillness, serene and peaceful. When I saw the two who were still, Jesus said to me, "It is simple, simple, simple."

I knew without the words being spoken that Jesus was saying healing is to be simple. When a patient comes to you, they are looking **Healing is to be simple.** for a cure and an end to the symptoms they're experiencing. And in my vision, Jesus said that healing is to be simple, simple, simple!

This vision echoed what He has already told us — His ways are not complicated. They are simple. It is we who complicate things because we do not understand, and we're misled by that lack of understanding.

These alignments aren't meant to give you yet another complicated tool or method to apply to your life. Instead, they will *simplify your approach and release you* from the complexities and complications you have accepted without realizing it. The first step is to go back to the original plan.

GOD'S VISION FOR HEALTH AND HEALING

What you envisioned when you first chose your career and responded to your heart's desire — before things seemed to become more complicated — is most likely what God's vision is for you within His larger plan.

God's vision for health and healing is for no disease, illness, injury, or infirmity to exist in the presence of Christ *here on earth as in heaven.* As one whom He called to care for His children, you are designed to be a vessel for Him, standing in the gap as a conduit from heaven to your patients. This is the role of a Medical Intercessor.

Your job as a Medical Intercessor is to bring complete healing through the partnership of your blessed knowledge and the

God's vision for health and healing is for no disease, illness, injury, or infirmity to exist in the presence of Christ here on earth as in heaven. As one whom He called to care for His children, you are designed to be a vessel for Him, standing in the gap as a conduit from heaven to your patients. This is the role of a Medical Intercessor.

Your job as a Medical Intercessor is to bring complete healing through the partnership of your blessed knowledge and the power of the Holy Spirit, by working in alignment with Him and letting His healing authority and power flow.

power of the Holy Spirit, by working in alignment with Him and letting His healing authority and power flow.

This vision is powerful because it is simple. You will come to realize how profound it is as you go through each alignment.

God wants to Release Us from Our Chains

In my visions, God showed me that if I wrote this book for you, it would break the chains holding you down (see Figure 3.1 at the beginning of the chapter).

The chains would break off, and the white coat would step out of the chair and rise above the fog. The white of their coat would become whiter, and their hearts redder and fuller, filled with the radiance of joy and love. Then, when the patient stood in front of them, still down in the fog, the white coat would interact with the patient, bringing them to rise above the fog and be healed and free from whatever pain or ailment they presented with in the beginning.

The chains developed as complications because we veered from God's original design for us in the vocation in medicine. You can make the decision to be unchained today by a simple pivot of choosing *whose vision you place your trust in.*

Becoming intentional about turning and pivoting toward God's plan will bring you one step closer to fulfillment and empowerment in your career. It's not a decision you make once; it's a decision you make every day.

THE DIVINE CEO'S VISION GOES FAR BEYOND MEDICINE

When you partner with the right *Who* — the right expert — suddenly the pieces start falling into place.

Part of the reason we were divided between the Path of Science and the Path of Spirit in our mindset is that we felt we had so many things to consider *apart from our calling.* Along with worrying about healing our patients, we found ourselves anxious about making a living, following the law, navigating business considerations, understanding insurance restrictions, increasing our knowledge, and having balance in our personal and family lives... and that's probably only part of the list for most of us.

Yet, God is the expert in all of those things, not just medicine. You have a partner with expertise *not only in true healing, but also in true prosperity,* so you can live a truly blessed life. You don't need to sacrifice one for the other. God is our true partner in all things. He is not divided in His truth. He is balanced among all of the considerations and understands them all.

You have a partner with expertise not only in true healing, but also in true prosperity, so you can live a truly blessed life.

In Jeremiah 29:11 (NIV), God says, "For I know the plans I have for you, ... plans to prosper you and not to harm you, plans to give you hope and a future." He brought prosperity to His people time and again. This is an area of His expertise because He knows the world He made and how it works. He knows what you need to prosper because He made you.

Jesus could heal the sick with miracles because He partnered with God. And His disciples went on to do the same. We can too. **You can choose to stay in the rat race man has created or go back to the original Creator of the body and the world and allow Him to be your leader.** You can request His specific guidance for the work you do for your patients. You can request your Founder, who had the original vision for you, to return as your Divine CEO when it comes to medicine and your prosperity.

He Will Lead You to More

He's not just supreme in His knowledge, He's supreme in the wisdom, and He seeks to impart His full Spirit upon you. In John 14:12 (NKJV), Jesus says, "Most assuredly, I say to you, he who believes in Me, the works that I do he will do also; and greater works than these he will do, because I go to My Father." This is His promise to you. Can you not promise yourself to Him in return? It's time to reach for true healing for our industry and for our patients.

I once heard a speaker ask, "Are you living an explainable life? Or an unexplainable life?" He continued, "If you are living an explainable life, you may be falling short of God's glory here on earth." That stopped me in my tracks.

Are you living an explainable life? Or an unexplainable life?

Living an explainable life means you are only living within the minds of man-made leadership and according to another human's understanding. On the other hand, to live an unexplainable life means you have tapped into the signs, wonders, and miracles that God calls you to be a part of.

You must *decide* to accept the gift He is giving you, in all its glory. Even when you yourself don't know where it will lead you. It's one of the most exciting decisions you can make.

We as humans, with all the knowledge we could ever gain, will never succeed at healing our patients like Jesus did. Even now, all the astounding discoveries in medicine and the level of knowledge that has been obtained regarding the human body are absolutely fascinating and extremely advanced, but we could not come up with the *how* to heal to the point of canceling or eradicating the disease or illness on our own. None of us humans can ever compare to the abilities of creating a miracle, as the *Who* can — Jesus Christ!

ACCEPT HIS GUIDANCE

Imagine Jesus as a CEO who has just asked you to come and work for Him. Would you do as the young men do within the Jewish education model and commit to taking on the mind of your leader?

When Jesus invited the disciples to take up His yoke, they had normal jobs as fishermen, tax collectors, and tradesmen. They had already failed or dropped out of their Jewish education. They believed they had no chance to be anything more than tradesmen and would never be able to follow the yoke of a rabbi. When offered a second chance, they chose to drop everything, including the control over their trade or lifestyle, to follow Jesus.

I heard an author reference this situation as comparable to having Michael Jordan walk past a budding basketball player and saying, "Come follow me. You can have my mindset and play basketball the way I do if you follow me."[5] I love that analogy. Imagine being that young basketball player. Wouldn't you respond by dropping everything and going with MJ? What if you, like Jesus's disciples, decide with all your heart to go with and submit to Him and heal like Him?

To many, submission can be difficult. Submission means relinquishing control and giving up the power to steer the ship and instead just be the vessel. As hard as it is, submission is something we need to understand and master to avoid the rat race.

Part of deciding to partner with Him and let Him steer the vessel is admitting to yourself that you don't have all the solutions, despite many amazing medical discoveries and advancements and the spirit of excellence you exude. You still need help. Like Apple's CEO, you must decide to be humble and accept that you have missed something along the way. Can you, like Gil Amelio, realize you need to bring in a new visionary — who operates with a much greater vision?

Become a Heavenly White Coat

The white coat traditionally represents a position of authority and trust. When a patient schedules with you, their choice to come to you builds trust and establishes you in a position of authority with them, in that they decided to submit to your professional guidance. They submit their problems and symptoms, and you recommend the solution, an accurate diagnosis, and a prescribed treatment plan.

When you align with God's vision, you uplevel your white coat to a *heavenly* white coat, representing His authority over disease, illness, injury, and infirmities. If you have already submitted to God's authority and partnered with His divine wisdom, you are empowered through His partnership — God is working through you.

When you exercise your authority under His authority, you can do amazing things, not just for your patients but for your industry as a whole. His guidance can help you heal what is broken. Working together in His holy name, you can achieve exponentially more than you could alone. Take that blessing and choose Jesus as your CEO — align with His vision.

When you submit solely to the authority of man, as shown through the illustrations of the two pedestals, you risk getting trapped in a rat race where limited healing occurs, and power and authority are stripped from you. *Who* you align with definitely matters.

Aligning with God's vision is the first and most critical step in becoming a Medical Intercessor who stands in the gap for your patients, believing the will of God will be done for them. With this new understanding of what He wants for you and what He wants for your patients, you can now choose to align with God's will in your practice, even in the face of multiple priorities. In the next chapter, you'll learn why your own heart's desire — your original excitement for the role God has for you — is a vital tool for staying in this alignment.

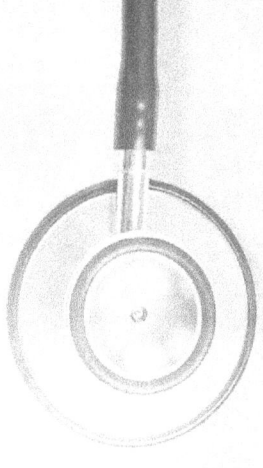

When you align with God's vision, you uplevel your white coat to a heavenly white coat, representing His authority over disease, illness, injury, and infirmities.

ALIGNMENT PAUSE

Reflection

1. Think through some of the day-to-day actions you participate in that are following man's vision and not God's vision. This could include rules, regulations, restrictions, or behavioral choices. List the things that are burdensome and don't feel easy and light at all. What do you think you can implement in your daily practice to help you align more with God's vision for your role in medicine as a child of God working for Him?

2. What do you think about what God showed me with the Pedestal Vision and the leaders who risk leading us away from God's divine plan for both Path of Spirit and Path of Science? Can you recall any leaders, programs, or organizations guiding your career in medicine that have veered from God's original design?

3. What do you think about God's vision for health and healing as being for no disease, illness, injury, or infirmity to exist in the presence of Christ *here on earth as in heaven,* and your job as a Medical Intercessor to bring complete healing through the partnership of your blessed knowledge and the power of the Holy Spirit?

Activation

1. Read the following passage from John three times and meditate on it: "Most assuredly, I say to you, he who believes in Me, the works that I do **he will do also**; and

greater works than these he will do, because I go to My Father" (John 14:12, NKJV).

2. Read the following passage from Jeremiah three times and meditate on it: "For I know the plans I have for you ... plans to prosper you and not to harm you, plans to give you hope and a future" (Jeremiah 29:11, NIV).

3. Ask God to show you anything within the scriptures that He wants to emphasize with you. Write down anything that stands out, and revisit it periodically throughout your next few days.

4. Speak this decree over your life: "I choose You, Lord. I surrender to You. Here I am, Lord, send me. Lead me, guide me. I choose to be Your vessel and work for you, and not for man." Create a visual of you in the vessel and God steering. Sit in this image for a bit. Write down anything you see, sense, or feel.

HOW IS THE BOOK RESONATING WITH YOU SO FAR?

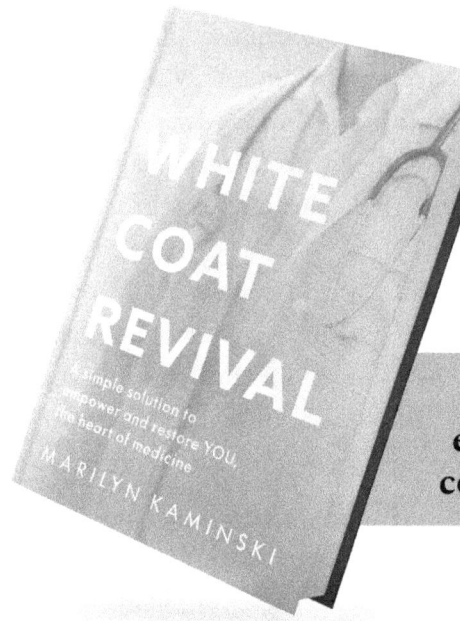

Have you felt the **immense power** it holds to transform the **medical world** as we know it?

Imagine the ripple effect this knowledge could create!

Help others discover this GAME-CHANGING book by leaving a review.

Your words can ignite A POWERFUL MOVEMENT!

WhiteCoatRevival.com/Book-Review

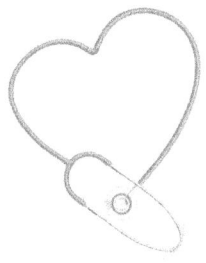

Chapter 4

ALIGNMENT 2: ALIGN WITH THE PURPOSE GOD INTENDED FOR YOU

For we are His workmanship, created in Christ Jesus for good works, which God prepared beforehand that we should walk in them.

— EPHESIANS 2:10 (NKJV)

Now that you've aligned with God's vision, the second Alignment is to align with your God-given, God-designed purpose. You were created for a purposeful assignment, unique to you. When you are in alignment with His plan for you, His promises are more visible in your life.

The current medical system has created a disconnection between what you were created for versus how you are currently being positioned in the role of healing. This disconnection is why we all feel that something is not right with the current medical industry as a whole, and it can also lead to constant stress and burnout, which can cause many to question our purpose, wondering if it's really worth staying.

White Coat Revival is written specifically to reduce burnout, increase retention of physicians, and drastically improve mental health. With those things in mind, throughout this chapter, I'll ask you to reflect on your purpose, recognize problems that create a misalignment, and learn how to align back to God's original vision for you. You'll find that once you're aligned with your purpose, your decisions will be tuned to His directional compass. You'll understand how to make decisions that feel right, without doubt and worry.

In other words, things will become far simpler.

PURPOSE ABANDONED

In the previous chapter, we explored many of the frustrations with the current medical industry and how we must operate within it. The results are devastating not only for individuals but also for the industry itself. The burnout and frustration that have engulfed the medical system have caused many to flee from the very purpose God has for them.

In a vision, God showed me a scene of a hospital (representing the Western medical system) burning up in flames while people wearing white coats were sprinting away from the building. That's exactly what is happening in our industry today — good white coats are running away from a destructive system and from the purpose God has for them. Sadly, the data confirms this. A 2021 Health Resources and Services Administration (HRSA) survey showed that only 57 percent of physicians would choose to become a physician again if they had the chance to do so. A 2023 survey showed that an alarming 29 percent of health-care workers, including 41 percent of nurses, planned to leave their jobs within the next two years.[6] How many other providers are thinking along similar lines?

This mass departure creates a double problem: Practitioners leave the divine purpose God gave them, and patients lose those called to heal them. HRSA projects shortages in all physician specialties by 2037, while millions of people already live in areas that lack basic care. The causes of these situations are physician burnout, poor mental health, and negative job and career satisfaction.[7]

Sadly, medical professionals are not just leaving their field; they're taking their own lives at an alarming rate that is much higher than the general population's suicide rates. This is absolutely devastating! In a report published by the American College of Emergency Physicians (ACEP), Dr. John Matheson wrote that compared to females in other professions and in the general populace, suicides by female physicians in the US are 250–400 percent higher. In addition, while male suicides are four times higher than those of females in the general population, in the physician-only population, the rates for male and female physicians are equal.[8]

THERE'S ANOTHER WAY

God has so much hope for you! He wants you to know you don't need to run from the purpose He has for you, and you don't need to give up hope. The emotional toll was never supposed to weigh on your shoulders. He wants to remove that burden from you and partner with you. His purpose for you is to be His hands and feet on this earth and live out that mission *with* Him.

When you are in alignment with your God-given calling and purpose, your days are easier, you have confidence in your position, and you can recognize God as a partner with you in medicine as a ministry. You can hear His voice leading and encouraging you, and you can enjoy working with your patients and fellow staff. You will feel settled and have peace regarding your situation.

When you are out of alignment with this purpose, however, things get harder, and they seem more difficult. It started out simple. How did it get so complicated along the way?

The answer is similar to what we saw in Chapter 3. It goes back to the same question: What is getting between us and God?

GOD'S PATH FOR YOUR PURPOSE WAS DIVIDED

Before you were born, God already had a perfect plan for you. As a child, you likely felt the heart's desire He placed within you. But then, as you continued your journey through life, outside influences made you think you needed to adjust the plan for some important-sounding reasons.

I have an illustration that I use in the ViaRayma courses[9] showing the path of alignment with God's purpose for us. I call it the Alignment Arc.

When God creates a purpose for us, He knows the beginning and end of our purposeful path. We can think of this path as the perfect arc containing everything He has promised for us if we stay in 100 percent alignment with Him and fulfill that purpose. An Alignment Arc in which we are 100 percent aligned with God, free of any detour journeys and traveling the Path of Spirit and the Path of Science as one, is difficult for anyone to achieve here on earth, but it is God's original vision.

However, though we have this path set within us, we also have free will to listen to other influences. The first outside influence most likely happened without our even being aware. Look at Figure 4.1 and observe the immediate split course that commonly occurs, causing us to deviate from the 100 percent Alignment Arc created when we chose our vocation. Many of us were instructed by parents or teachers to choose a career but then were not instructed to ask God what path to take to achieve that career. Instead, we were sent on a journey to determine that path from leaders or influencers in our lives — but not intentionally guided by God.

This immediately sent us on a split course — The Path of Soul (seeking science-based knowledge) and the Path of Spirit (seeking a relationship with God) as two separate journeys. Sometimes we hear the voice within us and are drawn back in, and other times we detour further.

FIGURE 4.1 THE ALIGNMENT ARC: THE PATH WE ALL COMMONLY JOURNEY ALONG.

DRAW IN YOUR DETOUR AND ALIGNMENT PATHS

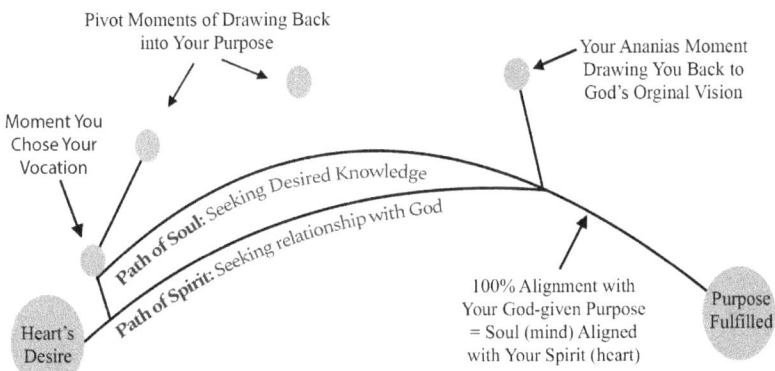

While you journeyed along your path seeking knowledge, other voices (even some inside your own mind) may have said to do this or that. Even though those things didn't feel right according to your inner sense, you continued to allow them to guide you, not necessarily according to God's divine plan for you. Over time, your original plan got fuzzier and fuzzier as other things seemed to override it.

When you don't hear God's guidance and only make decisions with your knowledge, will, and emotions, you end up delaying God's promises in your life. God is always with us. The connection is present, but you are not still enough to hear. Instead of listening to God's guidance, you process the decision only in terms of what you "should" or "should not" do based on influences of profitability, reputation, fear, or whatever other reasons you choose to weigh in the equation.

Remember that you enter the Tree of the Knowledge of Good and Evil when you process each decision within the confines of your own mind. Many of those mind-only decisions are based on your emotions, with fear, doubt, or pride often underlying them. This is not operating out of alignment with God's vision but instead operating from a disconnected heart's desire (your connection with God). That is how your own mind can lead you astray.

I like how Beth Powell, my spiritual mentor and one of my favorite people, defines this problem. She says that **too often, we leave our hearts behind and just live from our minds alone.**[10]

> *Too often, we leave our hearts behind and just live from our minds alone.*

We often might be following misguided leadership and traveling along lies instead of truth without even knowing it.

Misalignment with our God-given purpose comes from wrong beliefs and a misuse of choice. We can believe that we are destined to fail or succeed, but God really does give us the choice to trust and follow Him or not.

In your career, what things have led you to make decisions with your mind without considering your heart? Are you off track? What mind-reasoning are you most susceptible to that has led you off track? What might be keeping you from being 100 percent aligned with Him?

Do you believe you were created to fulfill God's promise here on earth? Can you see yourself in your God-given purpose? Ask God to show you what could be preventing you from seeing His guidance. Do you know He wants to talk to you and guide you even more than you want His voice and wisdom? He is a faithful and good partner.

I once again invite you right now to stop, acknowledge where you are, pivot, and ask God, "What lies am I believing about my purpose?" Just like we did previously, you can release the lie, replace it with truth, and create new neural pathways in your brain that change your thinking.

God has a path for your purpose. His grace and wisdom are available to lead you to your path, provide for you on it, and bring you back to it when necessary. He is your constant companion and is faithful to you as His child. You don't have to earn His help. It's something He is well-disposed to provide.

When you are out of 100 percent alignment with your God-given purpose, your days feel heavy, your calling feels confusing, and medicine becomes duty instead of ministry. You try to avoid burnout and fatigue but are unsuccessful. Your career might meander or take detours into dissatisfaction. You don't experience joy in working with your patients as often as you used to or expected to. But when you're aligned, your work flows with peace, power, and divine clarity.

THE ALIGNMENT ARC VERSUS DETOURS: AN EXAMPLE

The Alignment Arc for my own life hasn't been perfect at all. You can see in Figure 4.2 that I was led off track by pride, fear, and a wrong belief. These kinds of detours occur because, although God has a perfect path for us, we don't always stay in 100 percent alignment with Him. Our soul (mind) takes the lead, and our thoughts, will, and emotions risk leading us separately from our spirit (heart's desire).

As soon as we decide what we want to do when we grow up, we can start following the leadership of man and not the Spirit of the Lord within us, and we get somewhat off track. Our alignment is just as much a journey of learning how to be in alignment with Him as it is getting to the end result on the path He has laid out for us.

FIGURE 4.2 THE ILLUSTRATION OF MY ALIGNMENT ARC AS AN EXAMPLE

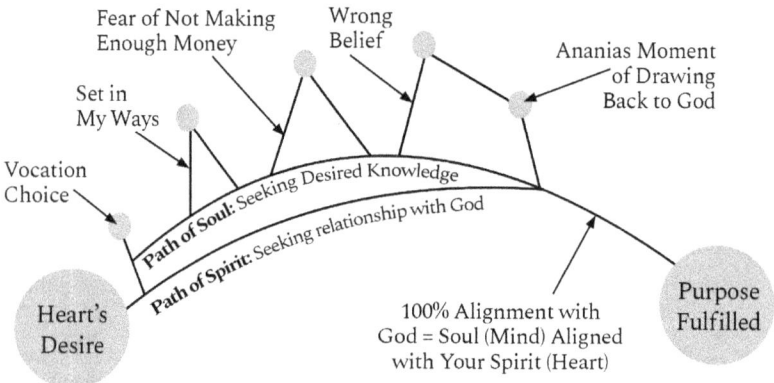

When you are traveling in 100 percent alignment with God, you feel joy and peace in both your home and work environments. Things move along with ease because His amazing divine orchestration has provided you with everything you need to travel efficiently along that pathway. Your thinking changes. You start thinking from the mind of Christ and access wisdom like never before. This is the real solution to burnout and lost purpose — your Path of Soul aligned with your Path of Spirit.

You were made not only to do the work God wants you to do, but to be supremely fulfilled and prosperous by it.

You were made not only to do the work God wants you to do, but to be supremely fulfilled and prosperous by it. It is part of our nature and an expression not just of who we are, but of Who God is, as our wonderful Creator.

ARE YOU ALIGNED OR OFF TRACK?

In your journey, how have your decisions aligned with God's purpose for you? Do you feel like your professional journey is aligned with God's vision to bring heaven here on earth? Is your mission to heal your patients flowing fairly smoothly, without too many challenges? When you do encounter an obstacle, are you at peace with the situation, letting God navigate it for you?

Or do you feel like you continually struggle to witness healing? Are you exhausted every day, feeling like many roadblocks stand in your way, creating a chasm between your mind and your heart's desire? Do you feel as if you are frustrated or hopeless a lot of the time, trying to think of what more you could be doing? Do you want more purpose? Do you feel you're just powerless, coasting along without meaning? Do you feel called to do more but have no idea what that is?

I'm assuming that you, like many of us, have at one point or another accidentally taken a wrong turn or missed an exit and had to backtrack to get back on the intended road to reach your destination. Sometimes it can take a while to realize you're going the wrong way because you missed the signs directing your journey. You think you are on the right road, and then something doesn't feel right.

You can only know that you're off track when you know what the journey is supposed to be. Once you know that, suddenly, other things become clear. You will be able to reflect on your journey in the Alignment Pause at the end of this chapter. I encourage you to do that. And even more importantly, I want you to focus on the amazing blessings God gave you, even when you were detoured.

HIS PLAN FACTORS IN THE DETOURS

Being off track is nothing to beat yourself up about or feel discouraged by. God has already included your free will in the equation and knows that you may choose decisions that steer you off track. These detours are part of His plan too. He's kind of a genius that way. He knows you'll get out of 100 percent alignment when you use your free will to try to solve problems that come your way, make decisions that seem right at the time, or make decisions you assume you just have to make without feeling you have a choice.

Even during those times, God is always right there with you, no matter how far you journey away. His favor, goodness, and mercy still pour out on you as you travel along the detour. You may or may not feel those blessings during your detours because the unrest and lack of peace cause you to hunker down and take charge of your vessel. But, as you look back on those times, you can often see the many blessings that were still given to you even when you were off track.

God is always right there with you, no matter how far you journey away. His favor, goodness, and mercy still pour out on you as you travel along the detour.

On February 15, 2024, I was sitting in a conference chair at a God Talks: Wisdom for Business event.[11] During one of the sessions, we were instructed to ask God about our business and ask Him what His big dream is for us within it. I attended this conference because I was working in my husband's business, believing that's where God wanted me to be.

I had entered the conference room that day exhausted and burdened from being detoured from my medical career and my heart's desire and purpose, though I didn't understand that at the time. When I asked God what His big dream was for me, I squeezed my head with both my hands and begged Him, "Please don't give me a dream about window cleaning or internet marketing." These were the two businesses my husband and I already had.

That day, I heard God pull me back into His will and alignment with the purpose He planned for me. I heard God's strong but gentle and compassionate voice say to me, "Change pediatric medicine." The voice came from somewhere above my head, not inside my mind. It seemed so real, as if a person in the room was speaking to me.

Prior to receiving those life-altering words, I was on a seven-year detour from my ideal Alignment Arc. Working in my husband's businesses, I was misaligned with the purpose God placed on my heart. I moved through my days with less joy and peace than God provides because I'd drifted from my path due to a wrong belief.

My marriage was pretty good. However, I believed I was obligated to be a certain kind of wife to my husband out of duty. I believed I was there to serve God and to be submissive to my husband and give up my "selfish" dreams. When I left medicine to work with my husband, I'd felt like God called me to a stage in life where I needed to be a good wife and partner with my husband in his business ventures and goals, and to ignore my own career calling. These were the wrong beliefs I held that led me off track.

Even so, there were countless blessings along this detour. You would never think I could have been off track, but all the while that inner voice deep within me kept knocking, because I was not aligned with my purpose. A chasm was forming between my mind and my heart. I was operating from the Tree of the Knowledge of Good and Evil, making decisions from my mind and knowledge instead of letting God lead. I believed the financial blessing that came from my duty and obedience was the sign from God that I was on track, but it was just because He loves us no matter what decisions we make. His grace is sufficient.

GETTING BACK ON TRACK

That day in the Wisdom for Business event was the pivot you see in Figure 4.2, which I call "the Ananias moment." The apostle Paul, previously named Saul of Tarsus, was pulled back into alignment with God when God sent Ananias to Saul with a powerful message: "Go [get him] for he is a chosen vessel of Mine" (Acts 9:15, NKJV). Ananias said to Saul, "The God of our fathers has chosen you that you should know His will, and see the Just One, and hear the voice of His mouth" (Acts 22:14, NKJV). That was the moment Saul pivoted from persecuting the very people he was divinely appointed to save. Instead, he turned to Jesus, coming back into alignment with the purpose God had always intended for him. Saul eventually became better known by his Roman name, Paul, and he went on to write 13 (or 14) books of the Bible.

It is my prayer that this book will be an Ananias moment for you, when you recognize God pulling you back into alignment as His chosen

> *It is my prayer that this book will be an Ananias moment for you, when you recognize God pulling you back into alignment as His chosen vessel to bring complete healing to your patients.*

vessel to bring complete healing to your patients. A moment when you choose to pivot from any ways might also be hindering healing in the very population you are appointed to heal. Step into agreement with His purpose and plan and journey along your 100 percent Alignment Arc as a Medical Intercessor — healing your patients through the authority and power of the Great Physician.

This integrated alignment with God can happen within you, and it can also happen within the patient. For the sake of this book, we will focus on the alignment with God for you, but in Chapter 5, I will share an amazing story of what happened when a patient partnered with God even when the physician didn't.

YOU ARE A CHILD OF GOD CREATED FOR PROSPERITY

First, you must know and believe **you were created on purpose for a purpose,** and He has plans for you to prosper. In Jeremiah 1:5 (NLT), the Lord said, "I knew you before I formed you in your mother's womb. Before you were born, I set you apart and appointed you."

The Lord continues in verse 17 to say, "Get up and prepare for action. Go out and tell them everything I tell you to say. Do not be afraid of them, or I will make you look foolish in front of them." And then He said, "They will fight you, but they will fail. For I am with you, and I will take care of you. I, the LORD, have spoken!" (verse 19).

And in Jeremiah 29:11 (NIV) we read, "'For I know the plans I have for you,' declares the LORD, 'plans to prosper you and not to harm you, plans to give you hope and a future.'" God has plans for you — for you as an individual. His plan for you is for good, and for your good.

Ephesians 1:11 (NIV) reminds us, "In him we were also chosen, having been predestined according to the plan of him who works out everything in conformity with the purpose of his will." You see, your purpose is God's decision and God's design. It is at the very core of your being, your spirit.

Second, you will become aware that God planted a desire within you to reveal this purpose. God gave you this heart's desire, this calling. Most of us sensed this heart's desire at a young age. Think back to Dr. Samantha's story in Chapter 1. She recalled wanting to become a doctor as young as age four. I remember writing a paper in sixth grade saying that I wanted to become a nurse. How about you?

Why did you choose healthcare as your career? Is it something you were just drawn to without knowing why? Did you fall in love with anatomy and physiology in middle school? Did you love caring for someone who was ill when you were young? Whatever the interest or fascination, it was connected to your heart's desire that God specifically planted in you to reveal your purpose. It's all part of His great design.

Think back to your earliest memory of what you wanted to do when you grew up. For this book, I have assumed your heart's desire was for a vocation in medicine. Most of the principles in this book still apply to any calling. Go ahead and work through this process, whatever your calling. Since this book is meant to align you with God's purpose for you, if the transformation process throughout this book leads you *out* of the medical profession, it is still doing its job. Trust God, and trust this process.

God's vision for His people is to bring glimpses of heaven here on earth, and He does this through your alignment with the purpose He specifically made for you. However, as you learned in Chapter 3, God isn't some ordinary CEO. In an earthly company, you get hired for a position you're suited for. God's organization is different because He is not like any other CEO. He not only has a vision for heaven on earth, but He has also created the perfect and necessary role for His promise and vision to be

He not only has a vision for heaven on earth, but He has also created the perfect and necessary role for His promise and vision to be fulfilled by you. fulfilled by you. He designed you for this purposeful role, and He is the One Who gave you your heart's desire. It was all in His big vision.

GOD GAVE YOU A PERFECT COMPASS

Purpose is your divine assignment from God. It's the meaning of your life. It's what gives you identity in Him. Your true identity is bestowed by God. He made you in His image and then called you as His child. He decided before your entrance into the world that He would be by your side and would put a calling into you that would bless others while blessing you with growth and maturity.

Understanding your purpose will give you the key to navigate your journey while staying in 100 percent alignment with God. In the previous chapter, we acknowledged that we often have a misaligned big-picture vision. But now that you've chosen to treat God as the Divine CEO, you can keep His vision in mind as you make decisions. Still, how do you know which decisions keep you on track and which ones take you off track?

Purpose is also revealed in the intersection of gifts, passions, and divine assignment. It is discovered as we look at how God made us, at what stirs us up, and in a knowing that we are in the right place at the right time. Along with your calling or purpose, God gave you gifts and abilities. These often come in seed form, but as you exercise yourself to learn and do, you see these abilities blossom. When you are doing something you feel "made to do," that is a clue that you are in your purpose.

When your passion intersects with your talents and abilities, you are likely in the sweet spot of divine purpose, but as always, you should still talk to God about your assignment. He is your CEO, your partner, your source of wisdom and help, so ask Him to confirm your purpose when you believe you're headed to or in your purpose. He knows how to talk to you and lead you to peace and success, which are also good indicators of walking in your purpose.

The solution is simple: God gave you your heart's desire, a fundamental knowing of your purpose. It is your compass. It is the beacon He gave you. It's your Spirit, and it's within you.

> *God gave you your heart's desire, a fundamental knowing of your purpose. It is your compass. It is the beacon He gave you. It's your Spirit, and it's within you.*

We just need to tune into this God-given compass. What does your heart's desire (your spirit) tell you? Don't mistake this for your soul's heart, which can be misled by emotions or wrong teachings. Your spirit is that voice deep within that keeps calling. When you start listening to it all the time and asking questions when you don't understand what you are hearing, you will be able to feel which way to go. Your heart will tell you.

When you accept that God is good and that He made you in order to bless you and to make you a blessing, you are free to expect that He will also guide you in a productive purpose. He is ready for you to ask Him about your purpose. Right now, you can take some time alone to worship God for His goodness and then ask Him to show you what you need to know about your purpose. Give yourself some time to receive His response, and write down anything you feel, see, hear, or sense.

RETURNING TO YOUR HEART'S DESIRE

Are you beginning to see how you can continue working in the profession of your heart's desire with renewed energy and joy? I hope so. Whatever your situation, however you've been feeling, there's hope. If you've been wanting more from your profession but are unsure what "more" is, I can assure you, it's God knocking. He is pursuing you and drawing you into alignment with Him.

If you have been stuck in the dual mindset that separates or limits your work and your faith, you may be in the process of getting lost. You probably still have confidence, though you don't realize you're walking down the wrong path. Something feels off to you, but you feel you'll just make your way through. If this is you, keep reading. You could learn some things that will help you get back into alignment with your purpose, even though you didn't know you were going in the wrong direction. Wouldn't it be great if you didn't get too far down that wrong path?

On the other hand, if your hope for your profession is gone or almost gone, you may already have started seeking a whole new path. You may feel completely lost or even abandoned, with little hope of returning. I feel your pain. Please continue to read this book. God has so much hope to present to you. He is pursuing you and wants to embrace you fully with His love, pivot you, draw you back to Him, and reignite your purpose to care for His prize creation — the human body!

He is pursuing you and wants to embrace you fully with His love

Your belief in your purpose that God specifically designed for you is what will allow you to make the positive changes that bring you back into alignment with His path for you and align with your heart's desire. His ways are greater than our ways! In Isaiah 55:9 (NIV) God says, "As the heavens are higher than the earth, so are my ways higher than your ways, And my thoughts than your thoughts." God's ways are greater than we can ever imagine. Be still and know He is God, and listen to His direction for you.

You have access to God's voice. Be still and hear from Him.

God has big dreams for you. He has unique dreams for each of us. He doesn't put anything on your heart that He hasn't already planned out. When you receive a big dream from God, please hold it in belief. God will not show you your big dream and then put you on a hopeless path. He will show you, equip you, pursue you, and lead you with wisdom to a shortcut or the pass through of the mountain that you didn't even see. What you thought was a mountain in front of you is now under your feet.

I mentor many physicians and medical practitioners. One of the most common discoveries we get to in our sessions is that they have a big dream to impact healing through an invention, a business idea, a medical training curriculum, or a workplace strategy, but they feel it's impossible to achieve. They are traveling on a detour, not believing that the inner dream is a knock from God, drawing them into alignment for their purpose to be fulfilled. They often express to me that it's a dream for the future. That's a lie. It's for now. God doesn't put that in your heart for later; He puts it in your heart for now.

I love coming alongside you and making dreams reality, with the power of God's partnership. He is an amazing co-worker. He does it for you. It's so simple, but it starts with knowing that knock, that inner desire, is not to be pushed away. Answer the knock! Don't try alone to carry the weight of making it a reality. Partner with Him and make the impossible possible through the power of *co-laboring* on those dreams with Him. Be sure to check out my ad in the back of the book for my mentorship coaching program. I would be honored to partner with you and God to accelerate making your dream a reality!

Remember, God's vision is for you to partner with Him to bring heaven to earth, and He does this through you in the purpose He specifically made for you. God is our extraordinary CEO who knows just how to work with us and through us. He is the one who gave you your heart's desire, and when you are on God's path of alignment and in your God-given purpose, your practice can be easy and simple. God's thoughts just drop into your head. His direction brings a clarity so simple you cannot believe you didn't think of the solution before.

Align with the purpose that God designed for you. Align with His goodness. Believe He does not take any of His promises away from you. They are always there. He redeems you. His grace is free! His mercy is magnificent. Believe you are here for a purpose, on purpose, draw into His guidance, living a life filled with peace, joy, and fulfillment!

ALIGNMENT PAUSE

Reflection

1. Do you believe you were created on purpose for a purpose to fulfill God's plan for complete healing through you? What do you think of the idea that God may lead you to completely heal your patient and free them in a way science may deem impossible — through His partnership and power within you?

2. Revisit the Alignment Arc in Figure 4.1 or download the Alignment Arc worksheet in the supplemental content (see the ad in the back of the book if you have not downloaded it yet). Draw the Alignment Arc for your life journey and your vocation. Are you moving along two paths or one? Is your mind leading you, or is your heart leading your vocation decisions? Can you identify various times when you were in or out of alignment with God's original vision for your purpose? Where are you now?

3. Recall a time when you pivoted back into alignment with your purpose. Do you remember feeling peace, joy, or ease after you changed direction? Recall those actions that ignited a deep level of peace and abundant joy.

Activation

1. Speak this decree over your life: "*God, I know You are pursuing me and drawing me closer to You. You have blessed me with knowledge of the human body and want to partner with me to overcome all obstacles and heal my patients. I want to partner with you. You created me on purpose for a*

specific purpose. Lord, send me where you want me. I desire to follow your plan and your plan only."

2. Ask God, *"What big dream do you have for me? What does 100 percent alignment with You, look like for me, Lord?"* Be still and hear His still, small voice. Write down, without editing, everything you hear, see, sense, or feel. Don't worry if nothing comes to mind at this moment. As you keep reading and your thinking shifts into deeper alignment, you can revisit this question.

3. Ask God to show you anything He wants to show you; then read Jeremiah 1:5, 8-9, and 17-19 (NLT): "I knew you before I formed you in your mother's womb. Before you were born, I set you apart and appointed you as my prophet to the nations." ... "And don't be afraid of the people, for I will be with you and will protect you. I, the LORD, have spoken!" Then the Lord reached out and touched [Jeremiah's] mouth and said, "Look, I have put my words in your mouth!" ... "Get up and prepare for action. Go out and tell them everything I tell you to say. Do not be afraid of them." ... And then He said, "You will stand against the whole land." ... They will fight you, but they will fail. For I am with you, and I will take care of you. I, the LORD, have spoken!"

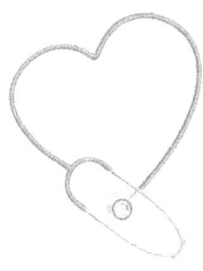

Chapter 5

ALIGNMENT 3: ALIGN YOUR SOUL WITH YOUR SPIRIT

Those who cleanse themselves from [what is dishonorable]
will be instruments for special purposes, made holy, useful
to the Master and prepared to do any good work.
— 2 TIMOTHY 2:21 (NIV)

You've aligned your vision with God's vision and your journey with the purpose God chose for you. Now, we are going to start aligning elements within you so your entire being is working within God's promise. In this Alignment phase, you will align your soul with your spirit.

In this book, your *soul* is defined as your mind, your will, your emotions — your knowledge, and your conscious and subconscious mind. Your *spirit,* on the other hand, is defined as your innermost being, where God placed your heart's desire in you before you were in the womb, and where the Spirit of the Lord is also dwelling within you.

Your spirit is your direct connection with God's authority and power. It was made new when you chose to invite Jesus into your heart (2 Corinthians 5:17, NKJV). I love how Andrew Wommack describes this new spirit as: *identical to the Spirit within Jesus.*[12] How incredible is that? This is the same Spirit that raised Jesus from the dead and the same Spirit that healed many! This power is now connected to *your* spirit. Its guidance is part of what simplifies everything else in your life.

Aligning your soul with your spirit is done by faith, and this process is called sanctification. Sanctification means setting apart, or in other words, aligning your soul-man with your spirit-man, which is how you are made new (2 Thessalonians 5:23 and 2 Corinthians 5:17, NKJV). When you grow in the grace and the knowledge of the Lord (2 Peter 3:18, NKJV), this sanctifies your mind, will, and emotions. Your thinking moves from soul-led thinking to spirit-led thinking — you literally think differently.

Take a look at Figure 5.1 for a breakdown of us as Spirit-Soul-Body, according to Scripture.

FIGURE 5.1 BREAKDOWN OF SPIRIT-MAN, SOUL-MAN, AND BODY

WE ARE CREATED WITH SPIRIT-SOUL-BODY
(1 Thessalonians 5:23, NKJV)

SPIRIT-MAN

Innermost Being — Heart's Desire Before We Were in the Womb

Made in Christ's Image

God in Us / Jesus in Us

Mind of Christ

Thinking from Our Spirit

Access to the Thoughts of God

Activated When We Invite Jesus into Our Heart

Spirit-Led Thinking — Influence from the Truth of God

Fruits of the Spirit

SOUL-MAN

Mind — Conscious, Unconscious, Knowledge, Expertise

Will

Emotions

Soul-Led Thinking — Influence Not from God

BODY-MAN

Physical Body, Cells, Energy, Brain Waves, Etc.

Recall in Chapter 2, the discussion about wanting and the importance of a co-laboring relationship with God. When you think with soul-led thinking, you are not co-laboring with God. When your thinking is spirit-led, you are partnering with God and allowing His power to work through you.

How do we switch to spirit-led thinking? That is the purpose of this chapter. You will learn to recognize the underlying issue, examine how and why it happens in your life, and eliminate it by realigning with the mind of Christ as God intended, so that His healing power can flow from you to your patient. This process will also prepare you for Alignment 4, where you will learn to completely transform the way you think about patient treatment plans and outcomes.

FAITH: COMPLETE TRUST IN GOD IS THE FIRST STEP

When we follow soul-led thinking instead of spirit-led thinking, the problem most of us experience, but don't realize, is that we don't truly trust God like we think we do.

Merriam-Webster defines faith as complete trust. [13] Do you have faith in God? Do you have *complete trust* in God?

For most of my life, I would have answered the first question about faith quickly and without any hesitation. I would have said, "Yes, I have faith in God. Always." There was never a stage of my life when I didn't have faith and *believe* in Him. I would not have thought twice about interchanging the words *belief* and *faith*.

However, the second question is different. When asked if I had *complete trust* in God, I may have answered quickly, saying, "Of course." And yet I know now that deep down, I did not have *complete* trust. I would have rationalized this disparity by saying something like, "Well, I have to do my part too," or "The reality is..."

There have been many times when I defined my faith simply as, "I believe in God. Yep, He exists. Yep, He took the weight of my sins, and I am so grateful for that. And yep, He still speaks to me and guides me. And yep, He has prepared a place for me in heaven. And yep, He blesses me often."

But now that I am back in alignment with Him, I can say that no, I did not *trust* Him with the impossible dreams or miraculous healings I used to pray for. I did not trust Him enough and have complete confidence in His will for no disease or illness or infirmity here on earth as in heaven. I did not trust *Him* to heal my patients — that was *my* responsibility, right? If I do my part, gaining the knowledge I need and positioning myself for patients to find me, then I will be equipped to heal them. Right? Did I really need complete trust in God to heal them? Can't I just trust in the knowledge I have acquired, or trust the extraordinary knowledge of my colleagues and medical team working with my patient?

Does Faith Belong in Medicine?

You may believe that trying to integrate your faith at work and follow God's will for complete healing is a challenging obstacle, and you may prefer to steer clear of attempting it. But those are all lies from the enemy. The enemy, seeking to disrupt God's amazing design, wishes to keep you from fulfilling your God-given purpose. The lies have been implanted into your subconscious mind and are blocking you from the peace and prosperity you could receive by being 100 percent aligned with Him.

You can believe and put your trust in your Creator, who offers complete healing and freedom from the chains of the disease through you, in partnership with you as the healing vessel you are called to be.

You can believe and put your trust in the lie that healing your patients is your responsibility, not God's, or in the lie that patients living with disease, illness, and infirmities are just a normal part of life. Or, you can believe and put your trust in your Creator, who offers complete healing and freedom from the chains of the disease *through you*, in partnership *with you* as the healing vessel you are called to be.

Western medicine's overall encouragement to achieve healing through your own spirit of excellence, paired with the expectation to heal within your own power, is getting in the way of achieving true partnership with Him. We chain ourselves to the lie of self-reliance because we want to maintain control and ensure we do things right, not realizing how substantially this lie limits hope and healing.

This misalignment causes your purpose, practice, and spirit to work at odds with each other, and your body and soul feel the strain. Your profession becomes difficult to operate in, and you can't do what you'd really like to do for your patients.

A tree cannot bear fruit that differs from its roots, so if you are rooted only in your own power, relying solely on cognitive processing, scientific evidence, and professional expertise, your outcomes will also be limited. When apart from God, you'll find yourself exhausted, striving to heal.

It's time to try something different.

ALIGNMENT 3

TAKE BACK YOUR TRUST

In this third alignment, learning how to place complete trust in God is the crucial step that will keep you from falling prey to the belief that healing your patients is on you. As extraordinary as your cognitive abilities may be, this belief that they alone will bring healing is the real reason we have a world filled with exhausted, frustrated, and chained white coats, as well as a high number of poor patient outcomes despite the most advanced research and technology than ever before.

When you trust fully in God's vision, you become a vessel, navigating your patient's healing together with Him — the God who heals.

Aligning your soul with your spirit allows you to operate from God through you, not in your own abilities, to completely heal your patients. **When you are aligned with God, the responsibility to heal is moved from you to Him.** You literally think the thoughts of God. You become the vessel for His will — simply transporting His power and His authority wherever His Spirit leads you.

When you are aligned with God, the responsibility to heal is moved from you to Him.

By doing so, you take on the mind of Christ and thereby exhibit the fruits of the Spirit (love, joy, peace, patience, kindness, goodness, faithfulness, gentleness, and self-control). You produce these fruits only through the Holy Spirit.

When you live a life by the Spirit — the same Spirit Who demonstrated His healing magnificence through Jesus and is omniscient (all-knowing) — you don't have to be exhausted. Instead, you can walk in love, experience joy that comes from the strength of the Lord, and carry a posture of peace. The fruits of the Spirit are not situational. Even amid the obstacles the medical industry presents, you can still live with joy and peace every moment of every day, no matter what patient situation is set before you.

Let me illustrate my journey from soul-led thinking, only trusting the medical expert for healing, to spirit-led thinking, trusting God for complete healing — a measure of faith.

A Journey to Spirit-led Thinking

Sometimes, it takes the faith of a child to show you where your own faith is lacking.

The morning of June 2, 2014, was a very bright summer day in Chandler, Arizona. My house was filled with two precious little ones who, as usual, woke up to face the day with joy and energy.

Unfortunately, a few moments later, the sun did not look so bright in our home.

My almost-two-year-old daughter, Deonna, was giggling with us in our bed when suddenly, her giggles stopped. She leaned back into my shoulder, her eyes rolled back, and her tiny little body went into a full grand mal seizure.

I froze in fear. As a Certified Athletic Trainer, I had seen half a dozen grand mal seizures prior to being a parent, but this was different. This was not the large body of an adult athlete who had just hit their head during a rugby scramble. It was my tiny, sweet toddler, whose giggling had been abruptly cut off.

Three minutes later, the convulsions stopped, and her little body looked lifeless and comatose. No giggles. No eye contact. Nothing but a breath and a heartbeat.

This day was the beginning of a nine-year journey that included seventeen grand mal seizures in seven years. Thankfully, pharmaceutical medicine came to the rescue. We were so grateful for the blessing of this medicine, but it only offered so much hope. Though the grand mal seizures decreased, our giggly, joy-filled, bouncy little girl was not the same. Something had changed in her.

When my daughter continued experiencing seizures and no causes appeared in her imaging and tests, the neurologist, an expert at a prestigious hospital, gave us no solutions other than to increase the medicine that was stripping away our child's personality. I knew she meant well, but I also knew there had to be something better.

Desperate for a solution, I started reading every medical journal article I could locate. Thanks to the internet, I could spend hours researching peer-reviewed journals while caring for my daughter. I found many articles, including some covering seizures and metabolism. I took notes, compared studies, and — aha! I was onto something. According to the research I'd found, it appeared that my daughter's glucose levels might be an issue, and she should be eating more fat and protein. I worked with her neurologist and a nutritionist specializing in epilepsy, but we only experienced limited results because of their skepticism about my approach. This was understandable since I was only trained in sports medicine, and they were highly trained in neurology.

Then, in 2020, our neurologist left the hospital, and I received a referral to a different physician who ran his own independent neurology practice. This was an entirely different experience. During our first visit, we spent 90 minutes with an amazing, compassionate, extremely knowledgeable doctor who spent so much time educating us, listening to us, and analyzing our daughter's history. He also ordered a DNA test, a protocol he requires for all his patients.

The DNA testing revealed a glucose transporter mutation. Finally! I had been waiting years for a legitimate, medically based answer for why Deonna had experienced 17 grand mal seizures over the last several years.

We started her on a keto diet in full force and a lowered dose of meds. No more seizures! Her personality started to become more vibrant too.

And then in May of 2022, our daughter had a dream of Jesus walking on water with her. After they came off the water, Jesus handed Deonna a big, swirly lollipop. Deonna said to Jesus, "I can't have sugar, but thank you for offering."

Jesus answered, "Now you can."

Deonna was thrilled and immediately came and told us about it when she woke up. She said, "I got so excited in my dream at that moment. I told Jesus, thank you, thank you, thank you! Bye, Jesus. I love you."

When Deonna was sharing this dream with us, it all felt so real. Deonna was so excited to now have sugar. She knew she could eat it. She believed it. But her dad and I had doubts. We downplayed it as a precious little girl's dream, but not reality.

Our little girl, now nine years old, had more faith than we did because we had intentionally taught her over the years to trust in the Lord with all her heart. And yet, we didn't realize we didn't have that same faith ourselves. That morning in May, we did not come into agreement with the healing Jesus had shown Deonna. We did not have the *complete trust* type of faith in God's will. So, unfortunately, she continued to take daily meds and eat a low carb, no sugar diet because we decided to not believe.

Why would we not believe? We'd already received other miracles. Only five months prior to Deonna's phenomenal dream, I was miraculously healed from an appendix emergency. I am sure my extremely exciting testimony planted a seed for Deonna to believe she could be healed as well.

It is curious to me now that, despite the miraculous healing I experienced from laying of hands only a few months prior, I did not connect our faith to the possibility of another healing miracle sent from God. Before and after the miraculous healing of my appendix, I truly thought miracles from Jesus were sporadic, few and far between, once in a lifetime — not something to put our focus on. So, when Deonna had her dream, it did not stir our faith to believe we were in store for another miracle. We had become shackled to our own expectations based on others' ideas or things we had learned. We trusted others, our own knowledge, or whatever else we put our trust in (soul-led thinking), instead of trusting the God Most High (spirit-led thinking).

Two years after her dream about walking on water with Jesus, Deonna dreamed about dancing with Jesus. When she had this second dream, I was much more attuned to healing miracles because I was getting daily visions from God, many of which you're reading about throughout this book, and I was actively focused on studying John G. Lake and his ministry.[14]

This time, therefore, I responded differently because I was now living a life from spirit-led thinking. I knew in my spirit at that very moment that she was completely healed. Only a few days prior to this second dream, I had read Mark 5:34 (NIV), which says, "Daughter, your faith has healed you," and I read that verse to Deonna. She has made that one of her favorite verses since that day.

The day we agreed with her miraculous healing, we started to taper her medicine accordingly and allowed her to eat whatever she wanted. After spending much of our effort to keep sugar from her for many years, we found it astounding that she was now sitting in front of us, eating a piece of cake. As I write this book, our daughter has been seizure-free, migraine-free, medicine-free, and eating a balanced diet, including real sugar, for almost two years.

What was at the heart of the difference in my response? When Deonna shared her second dream with me, unlike two years prior, I had *decided* to trust God fully instead of relying solely on my medical knowledge. Remember: Though I had believed for nine years she could be healed, I did not have enough faith to accept it the first time she dreamed about walking with Jesus, even though she believed it wholeheartedly. Now that my soul, mind, will, emotions, and knowledge were aligned with my spirit — the Spirit of the Lord within me — my response changed.

Deonna's healing occurred because *we decided to believe Jesus and not turn back*. We changed our thinking. We sanctified our minds and took on the mind of Christ in this area. We gained a confident trust in Him. God says, "Lean not on your own understanding" (Proverbs 3:5, NKJV), and that's how we have chosen to live since Deonna took her last dose of medicine. What an absolute blessing and journey of trust.

In Chapter 2, you learned that gaining the medical knowledge needed for healing is only half of the equation. The partnership with God is the second half. Trust in God's partnership happens when you switch from soul-led thinking to Spirit-led thinking. This concept of *complete trust* is the second part of the equation — it's trusting Him to co-labor with Him.

USE KNOWLEDGE WISELY

Our knowledge, which is stored in our mind and, therefore, within our soul, is a crucial aspect of our abilities in medicine, and it's important that we understand how to use it, according to God's vision.

To do so, we need to first understand what God says about knowledge.

The Source of Knowledge: Two Trees

The word "knowledge" is mentioned in the Bible 172 times. Therefore, we can assume it must be important to God.

In the Garden of Eden, God told Adam and Eve not to eat from the Tree of the *Knowledge* of Good and Evil, even though they were allowed to eat from the Tree of Life. He had a reason for that. The Tree of the Knowledge of Good and Evil leads to judgment — discerning, evaluating, and defining according to human knowledge and standards instead of God's — thus allowing humankind to make decisions in a manner we were never equipped for. When you operate from the Tree of the Knowledge of Good and Evil, you spend your life processing a huge amount of knowledge, data, and expertise to guide you to a decision within the limitations of your own human brain. You weigh whether a decision is good or bad, better or best, as if your knowledge alone will tell you the right answer, as if there is a decision algorithm you can follow that should always work. This method is burdensome and limited. This is soul-led thinking.

Applying this thought process to your vocation, as you learn and gain more knowledge about a subject, you feel more confident in your decisions. However, this reliance on the human brain alone to access that stored knowledge can lead you to get caught in the stereotypical 80/20 rule, where eighty percent of the solutions you present to your patients get pulled from twenty percent of your knowledge. This inadvertently leads to you developing and presenting limited solutions to your patients too often.

When you spend too much time analyzing the data, you risk swinging out of the Tree of Life, which is trust in God and His guidance. You are no longer following Him and hearing His voice and guidance. Too much knowledge-processing on your own can decrease the opportunities you have to hear His divine wisdom and guidance. It's so easy to operate from the Tree of the Knowledge of Good and Evil and weigh out treatment protocols based on the expert data, facts, and knowledge published in research studies instead of seeking the Tree of Life and allowing the easy and simple protocol to drop into your mind from God.

You are called to learn and seek an abundance of knowledge, but that is only one half of the equation of God's plan for you. You are not called to process millions of bits of information on your own. But rather, you are instructed to live as one with your Father and partner with Him and operate from Spirit-led thinking.

Knowledge Is Still a Blessing

When He blessed your journey with all this grand knowledge and expertise, He left room for you to partner with Him through that knowledge.

God is very clear in that He blessed you with knowledge. He gave you a heart's desire and a purpose to care for the human body. When He blessed your journey with all this grand knowledge and expertise, He left room for you to partner with Him through that knowledge. We will discuss this in much greater detail in Chapter 9.

Knowledge only becomes a problem or an obstacle to hearing God's will when you forget about His power and the gift of the mind of Christ within you. Instead, you need to invite God in at the beginning and ask Him to use your knowledge as His tool to give you much greater insight than you might have otherwise.

Some of us have never thought about this. You may have attempted to integrate Him into your workday, but not many of us have understood our role under our Divine CEO as the vessel He called us to be, so He could flow through us to our patients. Our job is to stand in the gap and become the Medical Intercessor God called us to be for our patients.

Trust Your CEO's Expertise Too

Let's go back to the idea of God as your CEO. If you were working for a company, and your CEO was a well-respected visionary with an amazing track record, great knowledge and expertise, and a long string of successes under their belt, would you question their vision? Would you try to hijack their vision and plan and not work with the team and processes they have provided? Would you defy the CEO by trying to control the outcomes, despite having way less experience implementing such a vast plan?

It's not very commendable. And yet, this is exactly what we do every time we choose not to partner with the Holy Spirit to heal our patients when we need to. God's vision is vast — something we have rarely experienced within our profession. We should trust His way, as His ways are greater than our ways.

Remember: It's about *who*, not *how*. Let the right *Who* come in and lead you. He will send you all kinds of guidance, knowledge, modalities, and even people, as well as His own omniscient wisdom, *if you allow Him to*. This alignment with Him will offer complete healing to your patient, not just managed symptoms or limited hope.

He doesn't want you to just be an order-taker. He expects you to be a co-creator. He does want you to listen and gain discernment for when you need to let Him tell you important things or bring others in to help you achieve the best results. Those others can include your patients.

My daughter Deonna took charge of her own healing by going straight to Jesus. She took direction right from Him. Her faith was pure, and it gave her hope beyond what her physician or I could provide. That's a miracle in itself! Your patients are not helpless victims. Let them participate in their own healing with you and directly with God. You might be amazed at the results.

Keep in mind that God is the true guide in this whole process. I'm just telling you what He's telling me, to the best of my ability. Ultimately, He's showing me how to help you find Him more clearly as your guide. As I said previously, my hope is that this book is written as His instrument to nudge you back into alignment with Him and His plans for you — specifically, how to align with Him in healthcare.

When you are aligned, your purpose, practice, and spirit are working in unity. You feel a sense of peace. You know that as a co-creator working in a relationship with God, you are able to provide your patients with hope and healing. You don't feel at odds with the world around you because God shows you the way through and around obstacles. And the best way to know? You think differently.

Aligned, your purpose, practice, and spirit are working in unity.

The solution is an intentional partnership with the mind of Christ — accessing your extraordinary knowledge while partnering with the Spirit of Life.

I hope you see that as you renew your mind (soul) to God's ways, you can have the confident trust in God that brings wonderful blessings to your patients and also removes so many burdens from your work. God doesn't expect you to grind away in labor for Him — quite the opposite.

HOW TO ALIGN YOUR SOUL

One way to proactively train our souls is by letting God's Word work in us. We read the Bible, letting it change and equip us, making us fit to do good work in our lives. Second Timothy 3:16-17 (NKJV) puts it this way: "All Scripture is given by inspiration of God, and is profitable for doctrine, for reproof, for correction, for instruction in righteousness, that the man of God may be complete, thoroughly equipped for every good work." Jesus prayed to God the Father concerning His followers in John 17:17 (NKJV), "Sanctify them by Your truth. Your word is truth." And, Romans 12:2 (NKJV) directs us to "not be conformed to this world, but be transformed by the renewing of your mind, that you may prove what is that good and acceptable and perfect will of God."

The word "prove" means to exhibit or prove out. When we change our minds to align with God, our actions change to line up with His good will. Let's put God's thoughts in our minds by reading or listening to His Word so He can change us from the inside out.

We also need to defend our souls from pollution and misleading thoughts. We should be "casting down arguments and every high thing that exalts itself against the knowledge of God, bringing every thought into captivity to the obedience of Christ" (2 Corinthians 10:5, NKJV). We can and should capture any thoughts that come into our souls or any belief or tendency we notice in ourselves that is contrary to God's ways of life, peace, righteousness, hope, and love. This is why it is important to ask God about any lies you may be operating from. The removal of lies from our thinking is a vital step in transitioning to spirit-led thinking.

It is a worthy endeavor to defend our souls, and we don't have to do this alone. God is our Helper even in this. Go ahead and ask for strength and discernment to guard your mind. God is faithful to answer. Today, I invite you to pause for a moment and look up to Him and say, "Thank you for choosing me, Lord. Thank you for choosing me to be your vessel so I can go where you send me to reach anyone you desire to reach. Thank you for blessing me with this knowledge and this heart to heal. I want to use it to partner with you."

That is so amazing. He chose *you* to channel His love for another, for your patient to receive His love and His abundance of health and healing.

We are called to live a life by the Spirit.

When your soul is aligned with your spirit, the evidence of God's promises shows up all over your life. He has many

Today, I invite
you to pause for a
moment and look up to
Him and say, "Thank you for
choosing me, Lord. Thank
you for choosing me to
be your vessel so I can go
where you send me to reach
anyone you desire to reach.
Thank you for blessing me
with this knowledge and
this heart to heal. I want to
use it to partner with you."

promises for you. The fruits of the Spirit radiate from within you: love, joy, peace, patience, kindness, goodness, faithfulness, gentleness, and self-control. And in the presence of His Spirit, burden, frustration, and disconnection must flee.

When you live a life by the Spirit and partner with the omniscient One, you don't have to be exhausted. The fruit of the spirit is not situational — so even with the obstacles that the medical industry presents, you can have joy and peace every day.

ALIGNMENT PAUSE

Reflection

1. What do you think about the story of Deonna and her visit with Jesus that led to complete healing? Can you think of any patient you know or have worked with for whom you could start praying to receive an unexplainable, complete healing from their disease or illness?
2. Do you think the impossible can be made possible, and the unexplainable can fill in where science-based research ends? Ask God to show you a current patient under your care (or a family member or even yourself if you have a disease, injury, or illness) who you can choose to believe to be healed.
3. What do you think about the fact that knowledge is mentioned 172 times in Scripture, mainly encouraging us to increase in knowledge, yet the only rule God gave Adam in the garden was to not eat from the Tree of the *Knowledge* of Good and Evil?

Activation

1. Practice how to be still and present in a parasympathetic nervous system state, and ask God to connect with you during your next encounter with a patient who needs healing. For more information on the parasympathetic nervous system, be sure to download the supplemental content using the code in the back of the book.
2. Read this passage three times and reflect on what stands out to you: Romans 12:2 (NKJV): "Do not be conformed to this world, but be transformed by the renewing of

ALIGNMENT 3

your mind, that you may prove what is that good and acceptable and perfect will of God."

3. Speak this decree over your life: "Lord, I release the weight of responsibility for my patients' healing in my own power, and I replace this with the truth that You are my co-laborer in patient care. I surrender the responsibility and choose to partner with You. Thank You, Lord, for lifting that burden from me. Please forgive me for all the times I held onto control and didn't trust You."

HAVE YOU INVITED JESUS INTO YOUR HEART AS YOUR LORD AND SAVIOR?

God sent His son, Jesus, to live in this world and demonstrate His love and power, so we can all know Him. That same power that was in Jesus is in us when we accept Him as our Lord and Savior.

With His power working within you, **you will think and act differently.** This is a free gift we have already received; we just need to choose to activate it in our lives.

I invite you to pause and make this decision now. By His grace, God has already done everything to provide you with salvation and bring you into His family. Your part is simply to believe and receive.

Repeat this out loud: *"Jesus, I acknowledge that you are my Lord and Savior. By faith in Your word, I believe in my heart that God raised You from the dead, and because of Your divine plan, I shall become one with You as You are now alive in me (John 17). Thank You for saving me and pivoting me toward You!"*

Receive this Gift:

1. *"Let it be to me according to your word"* Luke 1:38 (NKJV). According to God's written word, you were made on purpose for a purpose to do greater works than Jesus. You were called into a vocation of healing, so go heal.

2. *"Therefore, I tell you, whatever you ask in prayer, believe that you have received it, and it will be yours"* Mark 11:24 *(ESV)*. The biggest obstacle is unbelief. You have to first believe you can receive it prior to seeing it. Can you visualize and see yourself in a co-laboring relationship with God? If you cannot imagine a clear image of living a life in partnership with Him, pause and ask God what obstacle is preventing you from receiving it?

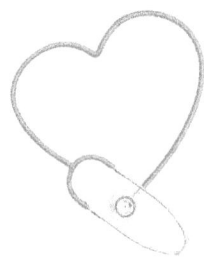

Chapter 6

ALIGNMENT 4: ALIGN YOUR EXPECTATION WITH THE GOD OF ALL HOPE

I pray that God, the source of hope, will fill you completely with joy and peace because you trust in Him. Then you will over-flow with confident hope through the power of the Holy Spirit.

— ROMANS 15:13 (NLT)

Isn't God so amazing? He desires only good for all His children. When you are aligned with Him, the interactions with your patients will be completely different. The day-to-day, mundane rat race that the current healthcare model creates will be a thing of the past.

One of the most important Alignments you can make in or-der to witness miraculous and unexplainable patient outcomes is to align your expectations with the God of all hope. In doing so, you will get divine-caliber results. This is far different from just praying and wishing for patient healings.

Have you ever expected healing miracles? Or visualized your patients' incurable diseases healed without a scientific explanation? In this chapter, you will see how that power directly affects the prognosis for each of your patients. You'll see how your hope aligns you with God to achieve His true will for your patients, versus what the science-based world believes is possible. The more hope you have for your patients, the more hope your patients can have for full healing.

GOD'S DEFINITION OF HOPE IS SPECIAL

The first thing we need to do is to define what kind of hope we're talking about. There are two kinds of hope, and which one you're working from makes a huge difference. So, let's look at the two definitions and what scripture says, and expand our understanding of God's will regarding hope in the categories of disease, illness, injury, and infirmity. Once you have this knowledge, you can vastly increase your confidence in daily practice. This is the secret ingredient for aligning your expectations with God's every time you have a patient encounter, no matter how concerning the prognosis.

When your expectations are aligned with God's, there are no limits to what He can do through you for your patients. Hope is *how* you dial up your faith.

Yet hope is one of the most misunderstood words when it comes to

> **When your expectations are aligned with God's, there are no limits to what He can do through you for your patients. Hope is how you dial up your faith.**

our spiritual growth. Many people think of hope as wishful thinking that looks more like a wishy-washy approach to divine intervention. We say things like, "I hope this helps."

However, wishful thinking is not part of God's way. Instead, we should be motivated by hope as God thinks of it: as a *confident expectation* that *anything is possible* through Him. Our motivation for healing should include believing in complete healing for our patients, even when it seems impossible. You are here to stand in the gap (Ezekiel 22:30, NKJV) as a Medical Intercessor between God and your patient. There's no room for wishy-washy expectations and no justification for them. If you're on His mission, you can expect He's working with you to get the job done according to His plan. Hope is the motivation behind the faith.

Can you see the difference between these two definitions of hope — wishful thinking and confident expectation? As you walk in faith and purpose, it's only natural to have a confident expectation if you are co-laboring with God. He is your partner, dedicated to your well-being. He offers you the ability to transition *out* of wishful thinking into thinking with the Mind of Christ, operating from the Tree of Life.

When you are aligned in this, you will think differently. Ultimately, hope is your motivation, and hope is the prize at the end of the race. This is why hope is the dial that turns up your faith. When you shift to alignment with the God of all Hope, everything changes.

HAS YOUR HOPE DWINDLED?

The fire to become a medical provider ignited in me when I had to undergo five knee surgeries in less than five years between my junior year of high school and my sophomore year in college.

I loved basketball, yet it seemed like nearly every time I stepped out on the court, I tore my ACL. I identified as a basketball player so much that dealing with injury after injury and sitting on the sidelines created a terrible mental and emotional battle for me.

By the time I had my fifth surgery, I was in college to become a nurse. I had taken some sports medicine classes out of interest, but my fifth surgery, which was for the terrible triad (ACL, MCL, and Lateral meniscus), became a huge pivotal moment in my life.

That was it. I'd had enough. That day, I changed my major to sports medicine so I could become an athletic trainer. I wanted to do everything I could to prevent another little girl from tearing her ACL and going through the same identity crisis I had experienced over the last five years.

I committed the next five years to learning anything and everything I could about sports injuries, female biomechanics, and the knee joint specifically. And yet, after all those years building my knowledge bank, something strange happened. My confidence dwindled.

And yet, after all those years building my knowledge bank, something strange happened. My confidence dwindled.

With all the knowledge I gained, I started to think that complete healing was much more complicated than I had initially thought it would be. With our limitations in science, I began to lose confidence in my goal to help a patient be completely healed from a knee injury and prevent a future injury — wishfulness took over, reducing the confident expectation I once had to limited hope.

When you made the decision to start your journey through medical education, you, like most of my readers, were probably confident you would someday do something great in your field. Perhaps you could eradicate a disease, end an illness, prevent an injury, or restore the cells of the body to complete health. I would bet that you didn't begin your journey in medicine believing those outcomes were just wishful thinking.

Then you got a reality check.

What did yours look like? Whether the transition happened as early as in your first semester of college or five years into your profession, I'm betting that at some point, your hope deteriorated into wishful thinking, and the confident expectation fizzled away.

In a way, it's understandable. When mine happened a few years after graduating from my master's program, I had finished seven years of college courses, and not once did I receive a message that complete healing, free from disease, illness, injury, or infirmity, was the goal. It's no wonder that from that point on, I operated from a wishful thinking standpoint, and I lost my confident expectation for complete healing. If your experience was similar, your reaction was probably similar, too.

It wasn't until nearly 20 years later that I had my shift back to God's version of hope and renewed my faith in miracles — and you can do the same, too, no matter how long you've felt your hope dwindling.

SEEK A DIFFERENT KIND OF KNOWLEDGE

When I heard God's voice, and He began showing me visions and dreams and connecting me to so many people who'd partnered with Jesus to reverse, prevent, and heal disease, my confident expectation returned. My renewed confidence came partly from seeking a different kind of knowledge — a knowledge of miracles.

You have to expect to see miracles. If you don't believe it, you can't receive it.

I learned that confident expectation is the key to healing miracles and transcending the limits of science and human knowledge.

You have to expect to see miracles. If you don't believe it, you can't receive it. Or, as Andrew Wommack says throughout his book *The Power of Imagination*, if you can imagine it, you can do it. Your imagination helps you see what can't be seen. Therefore, if you can see it and envision it, you can have it.[15]

God is limited only by the limitations you set on Him, whether you do so on purpose or not. If you remember *Whom* you're asking for help, you can confidently expect miracles of healing with His full participation, letting Him decide the *how*. This has been done many times before.

MIRACLES HAVE A PLACE IN THE MEDICAL WORLD

Scripture is a wonderful place to look for knowledge about how miracles happen. It is important as a Medical Intercessor that you understand God's will and are aware of the prevalence of healing miracles that take place in our world. These are not stories you find on public television or most people's social media accounts. Yet, they occur much more frequently than you may know.

One of my favorite Bible verses that has impacted my faith and my expectations is found in John 14:12 (NKJV). In fact, it's so powerful, I have mentioned it multiple times throughout this book. Jesus says, "Most assuredly, I say to you, he who believes in Me, the works that I do **he will do also**; and **greater works than these he will do**, because I go to My Father."

When Jesus said this, He was speaking to His disciples who had just witnessed countless healing miracles. In one of these miracles, Jesus touched a leper who had not received physical touch in years. Jesus healed him fully and completely. The sores went away, and his body was made clean! Jesus healed a woman from a blood disease that she had lived with for twelve years.

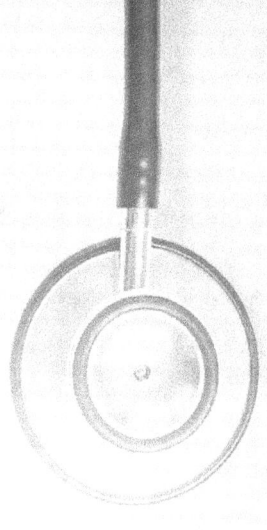

"Most assuredly, I say to you, he who believes in Me, the works that I do he will do also; and greater works than these he will do, because I go to My Father."

She touched His garment — just His garment — and Jesus looked at her and said, "Your faith has healed you." And she was healed. He told a paralyzed man who had not walked a single step in many years to get up and walk, and the man did. Jesus raised Jairus's daughter from the dead moments after she died. He raised Lazarus from the dead after four days!

These are only some of the miracles Jesus performed. And He told us we are to do greater works than these because He died, rose again, went to His Father, and sent the Holy Spirit here to partner with us. That same Spirit that was in Jesus then is in you now. You get to access the all-knowing, omniscient God from within you. Now. Here on earth. Wow!

> **You get to access the all-knowing, omniscient God from within you. Now. Here on earth.**

All you need to co-create with Him are two things: belief in the purpose you have been given by your Creator and the decision to follow His vision, His plan.

God Chose a Physician as an Evangelist

Did you know that Luke, the writer of one of the Gospels, was a physician? (Colossians 4:14, NKJV) Why did God choose a physician to write a Gospel? Perhaps God chose Luke because he wanted someone with knowledge of the human body to serve as an example for physicians to this very day. His Gospel writing includes many more specific details about the conditions and illnesses of those who were healed by Jesus than the writings of the other three Gospel authors.[16]

In addition to Luke's medical knowledge, he also had confidence in God's healings. This is an important example for us today. In Daniel 2:21 (NKJV), we read, "He gives wisdom to the wise and knowledge to those who have understanding." But we are also not meant to lean on our own understanding or to make it our complete foundation. To help us with that challenge, Proverbs 3:5-6 (ESV) admonishes us, "Do not lean on your own understanding. In all ways acknowledge him, and he will make straight your paths."

Today, we have a much greater expansion of knowledge and expertise of the intricate workings of the human body than Luke did back then. It's hard to gain so much knowledge and simultaneously set it aside to allow mystery to overcome our understanding. And yet, that's what Luke did in his time. We can learn from his example.

I created the ViaRayma Approach as an applicable skill development program to teach the skills to do just that — simultaneously bring God's wonders into medicine. The implementation of these skills shifts your patient goals from wishful thinking to confident expectation of complete healing.

Miracles Have Happened Beyond Scripture

Scripture isn't the only source of information on unexplained healing. During my research, I found many historical accounts of individuals receiving visions, dreams, and revelations from God regarding the implementation of God's divine healing here on earth, according to His will.

Oral Roberts

Oral Roberts founded Oral Roberts University in Tulsa, Oklahoma. He was attuned to God's voice and led by God and God alone. He led a profound healing ministry and was a well-respected man of God who influenced many Christian ministers, physicians, and authors, including myself. Oral Roberts University has a unique and iconic sculpture that stands 60 feet tall and symbolizes a message Oral heard from God to build a medical school. God told him, "I want a stream of my healing power to constantly flow out of this school through prayer and medical sciences, and I want you to raise up Christian doctors who will accept my healing power in its fullness. They will do all they can through prayer, and they will do all they can through medicine."[17] The statue has two hands that look like praying hands — one hand represents the healing power through the hand of Jesus, and the other represents God's gift through the hands of those who partner with Him in medicine.

Mayo Clinic

In 1883, the Mayo Clinic was birthed by a dream from the Lord to Mother Mary Alfred Moes. The clinic was intended for the only physician in the town at that time, Dr. William Worrall Mayo, following a devastating tornado that left many dead and many seriously injured. God told Mary in that vision that many would come to this hospital as patients from every part of the world, from every nation, and as we know today, this is definitely true of the Mayo Clinic.[18]

Catholic Hospitals

Catholic hospitals that were founded across the East Coast and eventually across the entire US in the late 1800s and early 1900s surely had the presence of God flowing through them. These hospitals were run by groups of nuns, and therefore were given the nickname the "sisters' hospitals." The nuns did not bring business or medical training to their work, but instead brought the presence of God, which equipped them to approach the challenges of healing by the power of prayer. Working in alignment with God provided a constant source of inspiration and gave them an untiring work ethic to see healings.[19]

John Alexander Dowie

Known as the healing apostle of the nineteenth century, Dowie earned his nickname in 1875 when the suburban town of Newton, outside of Sydney, Australia, broke out in a plague that ravaged the area. As a minister in that town, he performed forty funerals, and people were desperate for prayers to prevent any further deaths.

One night during that plague, two messengers knocked on Dowie's door, begging him to come pray for a girl who was dying from the plague. They said Dowie rushed to the house of the little girl, and when he arrived, he found her lying there, grinding her teeth and groaning in agony. Something in Dowie snapped at that moment, and he began to cry out to God for the life of this little girl. Suddenly, she lay still. When asked if she was dead, he replied, "No, she will live. The fever is gone." She was healed.

That was the moment Dowie realized the power of healing through Christ, and he went on a mission in Sydney, Australia, to show people that Jesus is the same yesterday, today, and forever (Hebrews 13:8). Despite many battles through the years, Dowie overcame the persecution and continued to preach divine healing. God's healing poured through him, thousands were healed, and thousands more were touched by the Spirit of God as a result of his work. Eventually, Dowie moved to the United States, where he healed thousands over the next couple of decades.[20]

John G. Lake

John G. Lake became a follower and student of Dowie's and was greatly influenced by his life's mission and healing methods. Lake also chose to partner with Christ and bring forth

ALIGNMENT 4

miraculous healing aligned with God's will here on earth. To this day, Lake's teachings have continued and have spread widely across the world. John G. Lake had 250,000 confirmed and documented healings across Washington and Oregon in the early 1900s over a ten-year period.[21]

These are only a few examples of pioneers in the faith. If you would like to dive deeper, you can research how they have influenced many Christians all over the world in how to partner with God for healing power. You will find access to a reference on him and many influential leaders in the faith at *WhiteCoatRevival. com,* which will guide you with knowledge of healing miracles, as they have me.

When you hear these miracle-workers speak and you read their books, you will gain knowledge of God's vision with regards to healing, just like you seek and learn science-based knowledge. You, too, will build your confident expectation that complete healing can absolutely happen through you when you partner with the Great Physician.

Miracles do have a place in the medical world. I can attest. I have seen muscle ruptures become whole at my fingertips, broken bones align and heal, an appendix emergency disappear, lifetime disease prognoses become a thing of the past, and even severe nerve damage restored. All of these were done with the combination of my medical knowledge.

Miracles do have a place in the medical world.

It is very important for me to emphasize to you that your knowledge is a blessing and a vital part of the equation. God intended us to gain knowledge through learning, studying, and getting degrees. This internal knowledge database exponentially increases when we partner with our Creator of the Universe.

God's message to me was clear. Being a Medical Intercessor is not about choosing either prayer or knowledge and science. I coined

You are to bring the science part, while He brings the Spirit part. This is Holy Spirit Medicine!

the phrase "Medical Intercessor" because, without the medical part, you are an intercessor. Intercessors are phenomenal prayer warriors. Along the same lines, **you're called to use your medical expertise** *as an intercessor for healing.* You are to bring the science part, while He brings the Spirit part. This is Holy Spirit Medicine!

EMPLOY YOURSELF IN CO-CREATION WITH GOD

You can co-create with God when you choose to live as one with Christ and be intentional not to separate your work from your faith. Remember: It's *who*, not *how*.

Let me illustrate this for you. In the summer of 2024, a few months after learning about John G. Lake and Andrew Wommack and many other non-medically trained Christians who healed out of confident expectation, I put my own confident expectation into play.

My family and I were at a water park when, from the corner of my eye, I saw my youngest daughter running. A moment later, she hit a wet, slippery floorboard, and her right shin did a pile drive into the edge of a large wooden step. Having worked on the sidelines of sporting events for eighteen years, I was well versed on how to react. Automatically, my brain registered the mechanism of injury in slow motion while I simultaneously ran toward my injured daughter and assessed the environment, her vitals, and noted the visual injury. I made a quick decision about triage and protective action steps all at once.

As I moved toward my daughter, I saw a deformity and swelling patterns that matched the mechanism of injury. Her leg showed all the signs of a displaced, closed, tibia fracture. I stabilized my daughter's lower extremity and focused on her vitals, being careful not to bring any fear to her mind and heart.

My old approach would have been to jump into flight or fight and determine the best course of action for stabilization and transport out of that area, but this time my mindset was different. I entered that situation with confident expectation that God can heal, and that I do not need to come into agreement with that injury as the final outcome.

I held this hope while stabilizing and assessing my daughter's vitals and analyzing the swelling pattern and the deformity of the tibia bone. Unlike my old ways, I paused and entered a parasympathetic nervous system response, becoming still and utilizing both sides of my brain simultaneously. I was then able to partner with the Holy Spirit and access the Great Physician, Who is sitting at the right hand of God the Father. I called upon His will to be done, claiming full and complete healing to her tibia, in the name of Jesus.

Still holding and stabilizing the tibia as I have been trained, I visualized the tibia shaft coming into alignment while the bone was made healthy and whole, as if the injury never occurred. As I stayed one with Christ in my mind and allowed Him to flow through me, the Great Physician's authority to heal was beautifully displayed. I watched the deformity disappear and the bones come into alignment while sitting in complete stillness with God. It was fascinating! I watched the little swelling pockets and bruising patterns recede. And I knew that my confident expectation of God's will for my daughter to be healed was in full effect.

She was healed as Christ flowed through me. His will soared way above what my medical knowledge alone would have offered in that scenario. I partnered with Him, and He met me in that moment to take the lead. I was just the willing vessel carrying stored knowledge and the Holy Spirit's presence.

My daughter immediately went back to having fun at the water park. In eighteen years of emergency medicine, I had never seen this. Amazing! I knew I was onto something about what hope for healing really can look like. This hope can be partnered with your extraordinary knowledge of the inner workings of the body for greatness.

The applicable technique I activated with my daughter's leg that day was one of the techniques taught within the ViaRayma Approach: *Medical Intercessor Visualization*. I operated with the hope, "If I can see it, I can have it." I didn't want to have a fun family vacation to be interrupted with a trip to the ER, let alone a kid stuck in a cast during the activity-filled summer days. I was standing firm in my confident trust that anything is possible with God, and He is the God who heals! In the presence of Christ, no illness, injury, or disease can exist! And He is my co-laborer in healing. The visualization invited the presence of Christ into those specific cells.

In the presence of Christ, no illness, injury, or disease can exist!

Keep reading. God is pursuing you for more greatness than you could ever imagine.

Your CEO Is Not a Wishful Thinker

Having that level of confident expectation goes back to choosing the right partner and the right CEO. His vision doesn't come from wishful thinking; it comes from confident expectation. He knows His purpose, His design, and what needs to happen for it to fall into place. He has *hope* for you. He isn't wishing for you to fulfill your purpose; **He confidently expects it.**

You can put Him and His confident vision into position to lead you, or you can put wishful thinking in His place. Unfortunately, putting wishful thinking into a leadership position won't get results. When you decide to work for the Divine CEO whose vision is the *confident expectation* of healing here on earth, then you get different results.

If you have chosen God to be the CEO of your life, His goals for you are that: You are commissioned to heal the sick and partner with Him.

Even Jesus Was a Co-Creator with God

Jesus, in His human form, did not have God's power alone. He partnered with His Father and brought His Father's will here on earth. Jesus said in John 14:10 (NKJV), "The words that I speak to you I do not speak on My own authority; but the Father who dwells in me does the works." When Jesus walked His earthly path, God displayed His magnificent power through Jesus's public healings. I imagine that all those who witnessed this power must have been filled with abundant hope.

Likewise, to bring the hope of healing to your own patients, it's important to understand exactly what Jesus said. We humans cannot provide the hope of complete healing without tapping into the source of the One who provides that. As we see from the scripture we just read, it is the Father who is in me that does the work. Therefore, we do not have the authority to speak healing into our patients without God's power. Isn't it mind-blowing that when we partner with the mind of Christ and allow His authority to dwell in us, we can bring the same healing that Jesus did? My personal example of the miraculous healing that I saw with my daughter's fracture is available to you too!

YOU CAN BRING HOPE TO ALL CHILDREN OF GOD

It is my prayer that the visions, revelations, and testimonies I've presented in this book will kickstart your own journey of seeking and expanding knowledge that will lead you to a renewed hope in the power that can flow through you to your patient.

Miracles only become possible when we act from a place of alignment with the God of hope, the God of confident expectation. When you embrace hope with confident expectation, you walk forward in your purpose, knowing you are not alone in it. This mindset is critical for healing and for becoming a Medical Intercessor upgraded to a heavenly white coat. A co-laboring relationship with God is what distinguishes the burned-out physicians from the Medical Intercessors. Medical Intercessors just position themselves in the presence of a patient and let God do all the work.

ALIGNMENT

4

ALIGNMENT PAUSE

Reflection

1. This can be a difficult chapter for some to take in. Much of what I discussed here hasn't been taught in many churches, yet it's been in Scripture all along. What do you think about miracles having a place in the medical world? Do you want to see healing miracles happening with your patients? If this is difficult for you to believe, take some time and ask God, "What lies am I believing about you, Lord, that would keep me from being a vessel of healing miracles?"

2. Pause right now and check out the resources I have included in the supplemental content (ad in back of book) and watch some of the healing stories shared there, so you can be exposed to miraculous healing testimonies. Taking in video content of successful faith will spark your imagination and your emotions.

3. Do you recall when you first set out on the journey to pursue a career in medicine? Did you envision being a part of eradicating a disease, ending an illness, or overcoming the impossible? Do you recall a moment when that confidence dwindled, and wishful thinking became the norm? How do you feel about shifting your mind from wishful thinking to confident expectation that your patient can be healed? If you are struggling to wrap your thoughts around this idea, please take some time with God and ask Him to show you anything that is blocking you from believing.

Activation

1. Read and reflect on Proverbs 3:5–6 (ESV), "Trust in the Lord with all your heart, and do not lean on your own understanding. In all ways acknowledge him, and he will make straight your paths."

2. Read and reflect on Romans 15:13 (NLT) "I pray that God, the source of hope, will fill you completely with joy and peace because you trust in Him. Then you will overflow with confident hope through the power of the Holy Spirit."

3. Read and reflect on Hebrews 11:1 (NKJV), "Now faith is the substance [title deed] of things hoped for, the evidence of things not seen."

4. Recite this prayer: "Lord, I surrender my soul, made up of my mind, my will, and my emotions, to You, the God of love and healing. I lean on you and allow myself to be inspired by Your perfect will. I choose to expect the impossible and know impossible healings are possible with the God of hope as my partner."

ALIGNMENT 4

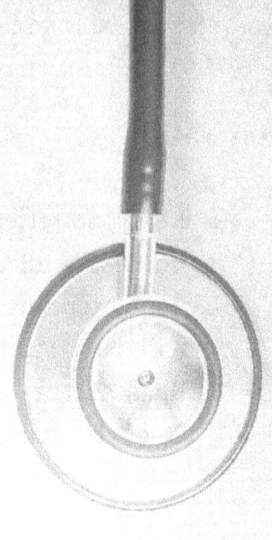

Impossible healings are possible with the God of hope as my partner.

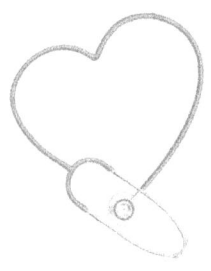

Chapter 7

ALIGNMENT 5: ALIGN WITH GOD'S LOVE AND STAND IN THE GAP

And now abide faith, hope, love, these three;
but the greatest of these is love.

— 1 CORINTHIANS 13:13 (NKJV)

ALIGNMENT 5

Alignments 1 through 5 of the 7 Alignments have to do with the preparation of the mind, while the final two are practical application steps. So far, you've reoriented within God's vision, reaffirmed your belief in your purpose, and aligned your soul with God — all of which have firmly anchored your *faith* in God's healing power. You then began to cultivate a posture of *hope* that is better lived out as confident expectation instead of wishful thinking. With this new mindset, you should feel more empowered to offer healing than before you started reading this book.

But before you move into the practical steps, it's time to address the most important internal Alignment: *love*.

Of faith, hope, and love, love is truly the most vital component to connect your God-given purpose to the previous step of hope for complete healing for your patient. **If you do not carry a presence of unconditional love, then all the faith you have in God's promise and all the hope you feel equipped to bring to your patient are nothing.** Love is the alignment that deeply connects you not just with God but with your patient. It's what allows you to stand in the gap so that you can bring them healing delivered from God.

> *If you do not carry a presence of unconditional love, then all the faith you have in God's promise and all the hope you feel equipped to bring to your patient are nothing.*

In this chapter, we'll explore the type of love you need and what happens when you don't carry it. We'll also explore ways to strengthen your love and understand better how it works in your role as a Medical Intercessor, or any time God calls upon you to be a conduit for Him in a situation with another person (or yourself!).

LOVE IS VITAL FOR POSITIVE AUTHORITY

As a follower of Christ called to the vocation of medicine, you have been activated with the spiritual authority to heal. In fact, you have been *commissioned* to heal the sick.

> *You have been commissioned to heal the sick.*

However, acting on this spiritual authority without love for God *and* love for your patient will, at the very least, *not* bring any additional benefit. In the worst-case scenario, it will create the risk of using your authority in an abusive instead of a loving way. Where abuse exists, it cancels out love — and vice versa.

When we act in authority without having love in our hearts, God is missing from the equation. If you possess a light affection or no love at all, you can't convey His love. Instead, you become a block, as if you've set up a dam in a river, and none of the water can flow to its destination. To see what problems that creates from a spiritual perspective, all we have to do is look at the medical system's limitations. These are often set up without love for God or the patient in mind. Without those vital elements, we rely only on our own limited, limiting power, and what we manifest shows those limitations.

Still, authority is necessary for our society to thrive. From the beginning of time, God created an environment in which one person would have authority over others: parent over a child, teacher over a student, president over the people, police officer over the citizens, mayor over the community, business owner over the employees, and physician over the sick. However, as we have also seen across different cultural examples, to exercise any form of authority without love is callous, oppressive, or controlling behavior. I'm sure we all can think of situations when we have observed authority exercised in the absence of love.

This is why it is vital to anchor your authority in love. When you do so, your practice becomes a conduit of Christ's healing presence and hope sourced from the God of all hope. Even your authority to heal is a sign of God's love for you, your patients, and the world, as well as an example of His magnificent power.

Paul teaches us in 1 Corinthians 13:7-8 (NLT) that love never gives up, never loses faith, is always hopeful, and endures through every circumstance. Prophecy and the possession of special knowledge will become useless in the absence of love. We are instructed to love God and to love our patients. We are called to store up knowledge (Proverbs 10:14, NIV). But, if you make this book about gaining all this amazing knowledge of what's possible and do not love as Christ loves you, all this new knowledge presented in this book will be lost and useless.

Love God in the Way God Loves You

When we say we love God, what kind of love should we be focusing on? Shouldn't we be trying to love God the way He loves us?

To do that, it's important to understand how God's love works. His love is a special type of love called "agape love," which comes only from God. This love is selfless, willing to sacrifice for others to achieve their highest good.[22] This love is the foundation that makes our spiritual authority safe, helps us use it effectively, and sustains it over time.

This distinction is essential to understand. Nothing I introduce to you in this book works without this vital ingredient. You need God's love flowing through you to bring healing to your patients, so you must attune yourself as much as possible to this type of love. We'll explain that more later in this chapter.

Love Thy Neighbor in the Way God Loves Them

Loving God is critical to deliver true healing, but loving your neighbor — your patient — is equally important. This love you need to operate from needs to be God's agape love too. Know that God's love for your patient is a love that is not limited by the world. It is a love blind to impossibility.

Your ability to hold this love allows you to flow the love of Christ through you to your patients. When you anchor your authority

> *When you anchor your authority in love, your practice becomes a conduit of Christ's healing presence*

in love, your practice becomes a conduit of Christ's healing presence; hope and healing flow from you because the love of Christ flows through you to your patients.

And that's the whole purpose of wearing the white coat, right? You want to heal your patients. The more closely you can align with Christ's love in this respect, the better conduit you will be.

Recall the story about the good Samaritan in Luke 10:25–37 (NKJV). The lawyer asked, "And who is my neighbor?" and Jesus answered him with a parable describing three different people who walked past the injured man, left half dead on the side of the road. The priest and the Levite chose to walk on the other side of the road and ignore the man because they believed the misguided teaching that if they touched an unclean man, it would be a violation of their professional status. But the Samaritan, who wasn't considered worthy enough to have a relationship with God at the time, had more love than the two who had devoted their lives to God. He tended to the injured man and took him to an innkeeper, whom he paid for the man's continued care.

Jesus showed that the good Samaritan was a good neighbor to the injured man because he chose to love his neighbor despite all laws and societal standards. God is glorified when we bring His love to our neighbors, demonstrating unconditional love with no ulterior motive. Jesus is the good Samaritan, and you are the innkeeper to whom Jesus brings the patients and entrusts you with their care. The relationship between the Good Samaritan and the innkeeper illustrates the partnership Jesus designed for healing — His compassion flowing through you without judgment, combined with your knowledge and expertise, and unhindered by industry regulations and limitations. Together, this partnership is what offers complete healing.

LEARN FROM YOUR TEACHER: KEEP YOUR EYES ON JESUS

God already gave us a gift to help us understand His love better, and to find the right path for love in authority and authority in love. That gift is His Son, Jesus. As a Medical Intercessor, you must keep your eyes on Jesus and look with admiration.

Let me illustrate this for you.

Have you witnessed a young, precious, joy-filled girl looking up and admiring her daddy? This admiration, displayed in that precious child, carries a love that drowns out everything else going on in the world.

There are many movies that depict an innocent child who is clueless about the stress their parent is experiencing because the love the child has for their parent has completely drowned out the trials of the world. Sometimes, the parent has experienced the loss of their job or their home, and they don't even have two pennies to pinch together, yet their child continues to dance and twirl and invites their parent to come run and play and laugh.

That's the same kind of love you need for the God who loves you so much and only desires goodness. We need to drown out the rat race of the world and be mesmerized by His will and His goodness. Too often, that feels completely impossible, but just like that innocent child, nothing else should matter. Nothing else should distract us from that admiration and love for what our Father offers.

> **We need to drown out the rat race of the world and be mesmerized by His will and His goodness.**

Our Key to Understanding God's Love

Prior to Jesus's arrival here on earth, man could not understand God. John 1:18 (NIV) says, "No one has ever seen God, but the one and only Son, who is himself God and is at the Father's side, **has made him known.**" This verse underlines that God manifested Himself through the human life of Jesus Christ. This manifestation is the key to understanding Who God is because it offers us the ability to have a relationship with Him and become one with Him in spirit.

In 1 John 3:1 (NIV), he exclaims, "See what great love the Father has lavished on us, that we should be called children of God! And that is what we are! The reason the world does not know us is that it did not know him."

The human brain could not grasp the capabilities of God's love and authority prior to observing a human demonstration. To this day, we cannot fully relate to the mind of God, but we can definitely understand Him more by observing the life of Christ. His selfless love shone through all His actions and words. Christ did not act alone to demonstrate that love. That love comes from a partnership with God. Just like Jesus partnered with His Father, so do we.

Recall the list of pioneers in the faith we discussed in Chapter 6 and that most of them brought healing as non-medical provider vessels — not medically trained at all. So, how could they bring so much healing? These amazing people brought the Spirit of Love — love that frees, love from God flowing through them. You, beloved, are equipped with knowledge of God's prize creation — the human body. Aligned with God's will, following His vision, created on purpose for healing, and motivated by His hope, how much greater equipped are you to bring countless healing miracles! This is why in John 14:12 (NKJV), Jesus says we will do **greater works than He did.**

Jesus didn't have medical training; He had a deep love for those He healed, and he had a partnership with God. Your medical knowledge, the compassion you have for your patients, and your desire to bring God into your day are vital for you to completely heal your patients.

I can't tell you how excited I am for the future of medicine! How fun would it be to go around freeing your patients from the chains of sickness? I know the more miracles I get to partner with God in, the more my joy overflows! You can have that too! However, I do warn you, none of this is possible in the absence of love. You cannot switch to soul-led thinking and think *you* have the power to do this. The source of this power only lies in Christ and Christ alone. We get access to God's power and His authority over sickness through the power of the Holy Spirit, connecting us to Jesus. None of this is possible on our own.

Our Key to Balancing Authority with Love

Jesus balanced His own authority with love as He taught His disciples, healed the sick, and helped the poor. Who could be better as our guide for this type of balance?

To receive His power, we need a relationship with Him. We need Him to infuse us with His love so that we understand how to bring that love to our patients. Without embodying the same type of love Jesus gave to all He met, we cannot ensure our authority does not become rigid and controlling.

This type of love also enables us to remain open to our patients' needs and desires. An open heart is crucial for our work in God's way as we heal our patients. Often, we must meet the patient where they are, not where we want them to be. Again, we come back to what we discussed in Chapter 2. If it's our *wanting*, we are missing the Lord as our Shepherd — we are missing the co-laboring relationship with Him. In my ViaRayma courses, I discuss the importance of co-creating with your patient *and* with God. If you find you are selfishly *wanting* your patient to be healed and they do not want that, it's coming from your knowledge and not the guidance of the Holy Spirit. But when you partner with God in this, He will lead you in each patient interaction.

I recommend that you visit the ad in the back of the book to join our community, so you can engage in more conversation about discerning wanting and heart's desire to heal each patient and how to hear God's voice and direction for each patient. Jesus didn't heal everyone the same way, and neither will you. God will lead you each time. It's not a systemized protocol. It's spirit-led thinking.

GOD WANTS A TWO-WAY RELATIONSHIP

The relationship between you and Christ changes over time depending on what you need. Sometimes your relationship is like that of a parent and a child. Other times, it's a spouse-like relationship in which you make decisions together. Sometimes it's a CEO-employee relationship, and He is the visionary Who assigns you to carry out the vision in your work for Him. And sometimes it's a teacher-student or coach-athlete relationship, where He puts you in charge of decision-making to see how well you do, and then gives you pointers.

No matter which kind of relationship you're experiencing, it doesn't work when it's not reciprocal. When a child is estranged from their parent, there is no relationship at all. A separated or broken marriage does not offer any of the same benefits as a healthy marriage. An ex-employee, or one who has no idea what the company's vision is, doesn't have anything to offer the CEO. A student who rejects the teachings of his teacher doesn't learn.

Only when love is present between a parent and child, husband and wife, CEO and employee, or teacher and student can incredible results be achieved. The presence of love innately brings two-way communication. Day after day, this communication brings the relationship closer when love is the focus.

The presence of love innately brings two-way communication.

I'm sure you've heard that we are the sum of those we hang out with. If you want a healthy parent-child relationship, hang out with your child more. If you want a healthy marriage, hang out with your spouse more often. Most of all, if you want a healthy relationship with Jesus, hang out with Him more.

That seems simple, doesn't it? And yet, sometimes we don't realize when we've neglected our relationship with Him. Life often distracts us from what matters most. And as we mature, our relationships change as they go through different stages of development along with our own ability to understand ourselves. Part of that development involves realizing when we're not being as reciprocal as we need to be in our relationships.

Ed Rush, my business coach, describes this problem very well. As he put it in one of his workshops: [23]

> Think about this scenario. Your son lives in your home, and he goes into the refrigerator daily to get some food. He goes through the food pantry and grabs some snacks quite often. In the evenings, he sits at the dinner table but says nothing to you. Then on Sunday morning, he comes into the kitchen, and without hesitation, he looks right at you and says, "Hi, Mom" or, "Hi, Dad," and he sits at the dinner table with an amazing two-way conversation. He listens and responds as well as sharing some emotions, but only on Sundays, not the other six days when he's in your kitchen or sitting at your table with you.

That example illustrates how many of us treat our relationship with God on a daily basis. We are definitely not "in love." We don't have any communication with Him throughout the week, and we don't acknowledge His presence in our daily lives.

But then on Sunday morning, we suddenly behave as if we had not just ignored Him all week long.

How strange is that? Sadly, we don't even realize that's what we're doing.

Just like the parents in Ed's example, God never leaves us. He lives in us and is right there with us all along. We're sitting at His table. We're eating His food. And it's not just in the kitchen. We're in His classroom, hearing His lessons. We're sitting in His employee conference room, being invited to share in His vision. We're His spouse, asked to share in decision-making. He's always with us, in all of His roles.

We just have to open our hearts and eyes to Him and choose to speak with Him wherever we are. Love Him like a little child fervently loves their mommy and daddy. Talk to Him. Tell Him your thoughts. Ask Him lots of questions. Be present with Him.

BUILD A RELATIONSHIP WITH YOUR SPIRITUAL SPOUSE

One of the most interesting ways God has helped us define our relationship with His Son is by calling us to prepare our souls as a bride would prepare to become one with the bridegroom. This may sound strange at first, but if you think about it, it makes total sense. We build our connection with Jesus over time, in the same way we would with a dating and marriage relationship. Dating is the first stage, then falling in love, then marriage, then falling in a deeper love as the marriage goes on. Those stages occur in our conscious minds as we gain knowledge about the emotions of the other person. We train our minds to accept or deny a relationship with them.

The first step in becoming God's bride is figuring out what stage of the relationship you're in and gaining knowledge about Him.

Are You Still Dating, or Have You Made the Commitment?

If you've realized you haven't quite made the full commitment to Him yet, that's fine. He accepts you wherever you are in your relationship. This is the time to think of yourself as "dating" Him. He is definitely interested in you. You know that because He called you to read this book. And He knows He may need to do some persuading. That's also fine — He's used to that.

Anyone reading this book who knew me prior to my late twenties will probably fall out of their chair in disbelief when they discover that I wrote it. I definitely was not living as one with Christ back then. When I look back at those days, it is very obvious to me that God still poured His favor out on me even when I was walking far off the 100 percent Alignment Arc of His promise and purpose for me.

My relationship with Christ has happened in two stages:

1. The initial stage, in which I had a lot of fun, but also quite a few moments of heartache. I was quite lost and made many poor decisions. I admired Jesus and thought of Him more as my comforter. I looked up to Him.
2. The second stage, in which I now definitely live, is a life filled with abundance and joy. This joy is much different and far more fulfilling than what I thought I had in my young and fun days. This is because I lean into Him as a partner and as my authority and have become one with Him. He lives in me, dwells in me, and now steers me more often than I try to steer Him.

What led me to the second stage of my relationship with Him was that instead of just seeking Jesus as a comforter, I started to fall in love with Him as the true authority and partner He is.

Love activates faith.

Love activates faith. For years, I continually sought Him, but it wasn't a love-at-first-sight kind of dating journey. It was more like one of those really long dating relationships where it took many years to determine whether I was in love or not, like a couple who dates for seven to ten years and then finally decides marriage may be the next best step.

In hindsight, I wish I had been more present in my dating stage with God and would have been able to fall in love at first sight. Instead, I had to sort out for myself what was important to me. Though I didn't realize it, I was putting what I wanted for myself into conflict with my potential love for Jesus. Like many of us, I would turn my "faith switch" on and off throughout my workdays and weeks to pursue my other love — my profession. This switch allowed me to juggle my two loves: my professional identity and my identity in Christ. See? We're back to that duality again. Once you see it, you can't unsee it.

I would find some time to read (i.e., skim) a few pages of many Bible-based books and would go through the motions of religion. I would read a few Bible verses now and then and listen to a wonderful biblical church sermon every Sunday to fill my faith's fuel tank. And yet, I was not building a relationship-based connection with God. Blending my faith and desire for the Lord with my core identity definitely did not happen until many years later.

The Dating Stage: Enjoy It

In the case of a potential marriage, the dating stage is a crucial time to learn about your partner. If this person is the one meant for you in marriage, then throughout this learning stage, you fall more in love each day as you learn more about how much this person shares your deepest values and has qualities you admire, which you believe will help you in a partnership through life. The more you know about yourself, the more you will see how to choose someone who will be a good partner for you.

The opposite can happen if that person is not meant for you. You would (hopefully) pull away from that person the more you learn about them and see how they are not compatible with you. Maybe they don't have some of the qualities you need in a partner or share some of the values you believe are important.

During this time, learning more about this potential spiritual partner can be both fun and educational. The following are some ways to date Jesus and learn more about Him.

Study Scripture

The first way to date Jesus is through the study of scripture. By studying the years when God was here on earth in the form of a human as Jesus Christ, we are able to learn about God through the personality and character of Jesus. The Gospels and the New Testament documented many moments of Jesus here on earth. When we study these texts, we learn more about God to determine whether we want to fall in love with Him.

I like how Simon Peter wrote this in his second letter to the church, instructing them how to love through knowing Christ:

> Make every effort to add to your faith goodness; and to goodness, knowledge; and to knowledge, self-control; and to self-control, perseverance; and to perseverance, godliness; and to godliness, mutual affection; and to mutual affection, love. For if you possess these qualities in increasing measure, they will keep you from being ineffective and unproductive in your knowledge of our Lord Jesus Christ (2 Peter 1:5–8, NIV).

Watch Depictions of His Life

I love the TV series *The Chosen*.[24] The producers of *The Chosen* have done an absolutely phenomenal job giving us visuals to accompany the words of the Gospels. The television performance has brought so much more understanding of who Jesus was and what He was like when He walked the earth.

I marvel at how peaceful and kind Jesus is in the series. For me, reading the words in the Bible without this amazing visualization created a gap in my ability to truly comprehend the love, authority, compassion, patience, kindness, and gentleness Jesus embodies.

The characterization of Jesus in *The Chosen* really helped me relate to Him on a much deeper level. This understanding has led me into a deeper love for Him in the past couple of years. You may find this as well, either in this series or a different movie or other performance that speaks to you about Him.

Ask Questions

If you're dating someone, don't you ask questions to learn more about them? Why not do that with Jesus? If you don't understand something, ask. Try asking Him directly and listening for His answer. You may need practice doing this, but after a while, it will come more naturally. We'll work on this more throughout the book.

Spend Time Together

Just like you would in an exciting dating relationship, carve time out of your schedule to learn about Jesus. Find time to have a lunch date, a dinner date, or a walk with God. Wake up in the morning thinking about Him and talk to Him. Ask Him questions, page through the Bible, and let it fall open to see what He has to say to you today. This is one of my favorite ways to connect, and I am so amazed at how the perfect message ends up right in front of me. The words are perfectly timed.

Ask God to show Himself to you through someone in passing and watch how He shows up. Listening to and singing along with worship music is another powerful way to spend time with Him. We are fortunate to live in a time of high quality Christian worship music like never before. Create playlists of beautiful worship music and play them in your home, your car, and at your work when possible. Sing! Sing loud! Sing out of tune — who cares? Get lost in the lyrics and feel His presence.

> *Sing! Sing loud! Sing out of tune — who cares? Get lost in the lyrics and feel His presence.*

See the supplemental content for access to some of my favorite songs and other books that helped me deep-dive into knowing Jesus more.

A COMMITMENT TO JESUS INFUSES EVERYTHING ELSE

The spiritual marriage to Jesus happens much like a husband-wife partnership in many ways. Like dating, it also goes through stages.

At the time of writing this book, I have been married to my husband for fourteen years, and though we run businesses and travel separately for work and engage in different relationships with different people throughout our day, we still move through life together as one. That's similar to what God is calling us to do with Him. He calls us to live life together and not separate Him from our work life. This togetherness is the ideal stage we want to be in with Jesus.

I do not recall how old I was when I began desiring to know Jesus. The relationship has always been a part of my life, but in my mid-to-late twenties, a switch flipped within me. I dated Jesus for five years before I fell in love. Then, the spiritual marriage began.

In marriage, we're still learning about the other person and ourselves. Everything doesn't magically become easier because we got married. We have to learn how to work together to make decisions. We have to learn each other's strengths and weaknesses, as well as our own. We have to understand what each person needs from the relationship. In my case, I had to learn how to balance my work and spiritual life to make enough time for Jesus. I had to see which decisions I was making that were prioritizing Him less than I should. These were all lessons I learned as I worked on our relationship.

Over the last two years, my marriage with Him has transitioned into a significantly deeper love. This stage is more like the agape type of love, unselfish and unconditional, where I know He is with me every day, in every moment. I've started to live as one with Him in my heart and mind all the time. This is when my soul and my spirit aligned. Recall Chapter 6 to help you align your soul and your spirit.

If you have this type of relationship with Jesus too, I commend you because I know it's only achieved through hard work. We all have our flaws that get in the way of our relationship with Jesus and others in our lives. Only through committing to work on your relationship with Him can you find your way.

As you deepen in your love with and for Jesus, you'll find it infuses every other part of your life and makes it better.

My husband and I like to lightheartedly say, "Thank God we love Jesus first and each other second!" We are quite grateful for that order, because without the agape love we have for Jesus, our daily *love meter* might dip now and then. (Like when he tosses his dirty socks right in the middle of the room and forgets about them for days, or when I decide to tune him out to have a lengthy conversation with a stranger in passing.) Thankfully, our abundant love for Christ gives us grace for those little moments and a reason to laugh about them together.

This infusion of love also extends to your profession.

When you journey through your days exhausted, burdened, and lacking peace, it's hard to carry the capacity to truly love others selflessly — it's difficult to bring healing to your patients. Healing comes from love. As we did with Jesus, we must fall in love with our patients. We must truly, selflessly want the best for them. Only then can our hearts be open to what God sees as best for them. And He is the best judge of that! He sees what we can't.

Love for Jesus Brings Oneness with God

This infusion of love from Jesus is the way to remove the dualistic mindset that creates so many problems in our lives. Think back to those two separate mindsets (one for your vocation and Path of Science and one for your faith and Path of Spirit) you considered in Chapter 3, and how they create a disconnect in yourself and between you and God.

How can that disconnect continue if you are deeply in love with Jesus?

It is just not possible.

An observable power exists in you when you allow God to flow through you, and you become one with Christ.

When you are one with God, you are also one within yourself. Only by truly falling in love with Jesus can you also fall in love with your patients and embrace your true mission as a healer in His name.

> *An observable power exists in you when you allow God to flow through you, and you become one with Christ.*

As you can see, to be a Medical Intercessor, the balance of love and authority is very important. Without love, your authority over your patient's health is nothing. If you want to exercise spiritual authority well, you must love Jesus deeply and let that love flow through your work.

With your love firmly in place, ready to make you a conduit between God and your patient, it is time to start putting your Alignments into action by learning to align while actively working with your patients. This will be useful in the next chapter, where you'll learn to work with a balanced mind and heart to expand your understanding so you can heal your patients on multiple levels.

Let God love people through you.

Do you see why scripture says, "love is the greatest of these"? Love God. Love your patient. And go heal! Ministry leader Joseph Z says it even better: "Let God love people through you."[25]

ALIGNMENT PAUSE

Reflection

1. What type of relationship do you currently have with Jesus? Are you in the early dating stage, or do you have a strong partnership? I encourage you to build your relationship with Him no matter what stage you are in. The more knowledge you have of the life of Jesus, the more you will understand who God is and what's possible through co-laboring with His love.

2. There is power in listening to Biblically sound worship songs. Additionally, specific frequencies of music activate parts of the brain to open a connection with the Holy Spirit. Do you have a good song list you regularly listen to so that you can feel the power of the Holy Spirit's presence? If not, check out my song list in the downloadable supplemental content to help you create a playlist of powerful worship music for your car, clinic, or home (see ad in back of book).

3. What do you think about the Good Samaritan story in Luke 10:25–37? Through this illustration, God defines what it means to *love your neighbor as yourself.* Did you catch the Samaritan's act of full compassion *and* partnership with the innkeeper to ensure the thief was completely healed? Did you ever think of your patient as your neighbor? A neighbor coming to you for help? What about the innkeeper? Do you think the partnership of both the Samaritan and the innkeeper was how the thief was fully healed?

Activation

1. Fall in love with Jesus! Do you currently have a morning routine to start your day off thinking about God? Try one of these suggestions every day for three weeks to create a new habit:

   a. Read a daily devotion.

   b. Take 15 minutes to just sit quietly in prayer with God. This may be in your car, but try to make it separate from driving.

   c. Or split the 15 minutes into: 5 minutes of prayer, 5 minutes of Bible reading, and 5 minutes of worship songs.

   d. Use a Bible reading plan, and read the Bible verses each day.

   e. Listen to worship music in your car on your way to work and soak in the presence of God. Don't think about your workday while doing this.

2. Read this passage three times, and each time, ask God to show you anything He wants to emphasize to you: "We have known and believed the love that God has for us. God is love, and he who abides in love abides in God, and God in him. Love has been perfected among us in this: that we may have boldness in the day of judgment; because as He is, so are we in this world. There is no fear in love; but perfect love casts out fear, because fear involves torment. But he who fears has not been made perfect in love. We love Him because He first loved us" (1 John 4:16–19, NKJV).

ALIGNMENT 5

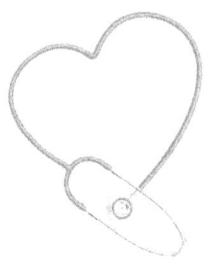

Chapter 8

ALIGNMENT 6: ALIGN YOUR MIND WITH YOUR HEART

*Do not be conformed to this world, but be transformed
by the renewing of your mind, that you may prove what is
that good and acceptable and perfect will of God.*

— ROMANS 12:2 (NKJV)

The previous five Alignments gave you a much clearer sense of your purpose within God's vision to prepare yourself as a vessel for God's love to pour through to your patients. Your mindset is more deeply attuned to God's mind in preparation for working with your patients.

In this and the next alignment step, I will guide you through what it looks like to apply this teaching in every patient interaction and to understand how to work under the authority of your new CEO — God.

ALIGNMENT

6

This chapter will help you align your renewed heart (your innermost being and who God made you to be) and your mind (your thinking) so that while you are working with your patients, you operate from the mind of Christ and access information beyond what you would receive if you were just working from your knowledge alone.

This chapter will build on everything you've learned in the previous steps, allowing you to draw from God's balanced, unified vision so you can see that what once seemed complicated and impossible is suddenly simple and clear.

This chapter is what shifts you from a stuck feeling to a feeling of freedom and a sense of hope that you may not have felt in years as your passion comes alive again.

A NEW WAY OF THINKING

In previous chapters, I mentioned soul-led thinking (operating from the Tree of the Knowledge of Good and Evil) and spirit-led thinking (operating from the Tree of Life). Soul-led thinking is thinking from your own mind, will, and emotions. Spirit-led thinking is thinking with the mind of Christ.

Your entire day is spent thinking — processing information and making decisions. And the traditional fix has always been the same: Add more knowledge. More data. More tools. Yet more of the same only produces more of the same. If we want different outcomes, we need a different way of thinking. I propose that medicine needs a new thinking style.

This chapter will help you begin to work as a co-creator with God and partner with Him to help the patient heal on all levels.

The Heartmath Institute has proven the physiological changes that occur within your body when you align your mind (your thinking) with your heart's desire (the Spirit within you).

When the heart-brain connection is more coherent, you have greater mental clarity, emotional stability, and better stress response. This alignment improves cognitive task performance, quicker decision-making, and fewer errors.[26] When we align our minds with our hearts, we enter the parasympathetic nervous system state that I discussed in Chapter 2.

In this state, you can *be still* and *encounter* God's still, small voice. This voice is God co-laboring with you and providing you the absolute best intel for your decisions. As Psalm 46:10 (NKJV) describes, *"Be still and know that I am God. I will be exalted among the nations, I will be exalted in the earth."* We need to first be still; *then* we can know.

This is Spirit-led thinking, operating from the mind of Christ, living from the Tree of Life that God so desires for you.

THE SOURCE OF THE DIVIDE

In Proverbs 10:14 (NKJV), God instructs us to "store up knowledge." In Hebrew, this means to lay up and treasure knowledge. When you treasure something, you keep it and access it with great care and respect the value it carries. To store up knowledge (in your soul) is to simply gain valuable knowledge. However, as you've already seen in previous chapters, when you believe you must access this stored-up knowledge on your own, you are limited and powered by cognitive processing abilities from man alone. Living in alignment with God allows you to access this stored-up knowledge through a partnership with the Holy Spirit.

The problem is not in how much science-based knowledge we have, but in the expectations of how we should be accessing it.

The problem is not in how much science-based knowledge we have, but in the expectations of how we should be accessing it. Our brains can get consumed with analyzing all the knowledge, data, and facts banked within our minds to determine what decision to make. This can become very burdensome, especially if you are trying to beat the odds of the 80/20 rule and not jump into an easy answer, but instead, think outside of the box for some of your patient solutions.

I believe God instructed us to store up knowledge and then lean on Him for assessment and interpretation. His divine wisdom can not only save you a lot of time, frustration, and energy, but it can also guide you to access the exact correct knowledge to reference at the right time for the right patient. Plus, it leaves room for Him to drop something in your mind you didn't previously understand.

In our profession, there's a dangerous temptation to believe, whether because of our education or assumptions, that when dealing with the sick or injured, *we* must fix the situation. Additionally, we are taught to hunker down and learn about every possible diagnosis and treatment option according to what research has proven to be true. And if we do, then *we'll* have the solution stored in our brains — or at least we'll have knowledge of a nearby resource to quickly reference and execute.

In other words, we feel (or have been taught) that our knowledge alone is the only key to helping the patient. If we believe this lie, then the limitations of our knowledge, along with the limitations of our current system in general, are allowed to dictate how we work with our patients and how successful our outcomes can be. This lie is what creates heavily burdened, exhausted, isolated, and heartbroken white coats. To reference the illustration from Chapter 2, the weight of responsibility for your patient's healing is just another chain holding you hostage in the fog, helpless in the presence of your patient.

The Wisdom Pyramid

God is in the business of multiplication. He is the *Who,* not the *how,* in improving decision-making. His partnership doesn't just slightly help; it exponentially helps you. His divine wisdom is the part of the equation that creates better results with less effort and allows you to receive the exact solution at the exact right time.

Ed Rush illustrates this best at every one of his God Talk events with *The Wisdom Pyramid* shown in Figure 8.1. When we partner with God and receive His divine wisdom, it's only one percent effort from us with a 99 percent result. Compare that to when we use our knowledge, which is 20 percent effort with only an 80 percent result.

FIGURE 8.1 ED RUSH'S THE WISDOM PYRAMID[27]

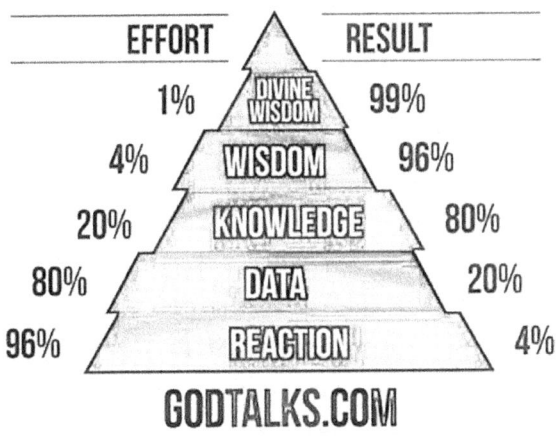

The Wisdom Pyramid illustrates the increased effort that comes with data and knowledge compared to partnering with God. God blessed you with your extraordinary knowledge so you could partner with Him — not so you could process it yourself. As we've already explored, that's why He warned Adam and Eve against eating from the Tree of the Knowledge of Good and Evil. When you process your own knowledge and solve problems on your own, it takes so much energy for limited results, and neither of those is God's plan. He wants you to be overflowing with joy and patients to be completely healed!

When you understand it's a false belief that you're singularly responsible for the decisions you make, you take the first step toward undoing the damage of this belief. And as we have discussed, that understanding goes back to one key fact: It is not *how*, it is *who*.

> **When you let God (Who) partner with you to provide the solutions and not rely only on your own mind (how), you offer an abundance of hope to your patients.**

When you let God (*Who*) partner with you to provide the solutions and not rely only on your own mind (*how*), you offer an abundance of hope to your patients.

HOW A MEDICAL INTERCESSOR WORKS

As you have noticed, I've included the term *Medical Intercessor* multiple times throughout this book. I chose this language to describe you in the role of medicine connected to God — other terms could be *a praying physician,* or *Holy Spirit medicine* or *faith-integrated medicine*, or however you would like to describe it. A Medical Intercessor is one who intentionally brings God into medicine, walking in their God-given purpose, standing in the Gap believing for complete healing for their patient and flowing the love of Christ as God's vessel — a spirit-filled love that frees their patient from sickness. This is true partnership with God in the exam room. This is the whole reason for this book: to upgrade you to a heavenly white coat as you stand in authority over disease, illness, injury, and infirmity.

When we lay up our knowledge and partner with Him, we allow God to pour information into your mind. It's a very different way of thinking that gets very different results.

As I've mentioned, while writing this book, God sent me one person after another to help me understand the message God was illustrating to me in the various visions and dreams about science and Spirit pathways. One of the most fascinating encounters was with my friend Aiden, whose case is a great example of how a Medical Intercessor approach can help when the traditional medical approach fails to offer viable solutions.

Aiden had debilitating pain throughout his back and hip due to a 40-year history of knee surgeries, hip problems, and low back issues. Due to his extensive health history, Aiden wanted to be sure to go to the best orthopedic surgeon to treat his pain. As a physician himself, Aiden spent a lot of time researching which surgeon he should work with. He knew his lengthy history and complicated case would require an experienced and advanced thinker, someone known for thinking outside the box and who was highly recommended.

Aiden had already had 15 knee surgeries on his right knee, including the insertion of various knee-replacement hardware. This led to his right leg being significantly longer than his left leg. This leg length discrepancy had created functional scoliosis in his lumbar spine over the years, placing an abundant amount of stress on the nerves in his low back and contributing to the daily nerve pain Aiden had been experiencing.

After he found his ideal surgeon, Aiden had to wait quite a bit of time to get an appointment. With his extensive amount of nerve pain, he was eagerly awaiting a touch of *neighborly* love and had much hope for the pain relief that this surgeon could offer him in the near future.

ALIGNMENT 6

The day of his appointment, the physician entered the room, gathered some health history, and, without much consideration, offered one solution: surgery on Aiden's good knee to add a spacer in the bone to realign his back by making his legs the same length. The surgeon recognized that the severe difference in leg length was the underlying issue causing the intense nerve pain throughout Aiden's hip and back.

Of course, as the God of orchestration would have it, Aiden and I had recently met, and I'd shared my vision of aligning doctors with God to produce better patient outcomes. So, when this surgeon offered him only one solution — an extreme solution, mind you — Aiden started wondering if maybe there could be another way.

Aiden and I had coffee together shortly after he'd visited his surgeon, and after telling me about the experience, he said, "I'd really like another option. I am intrigued by what you are teaching about partnering with God and better patient outcomes. It seems crazy to have surgery on my healthy leg. The solution makes sense, but it's a bit extreme."

Hearing this, my heart moved with great compassion, and I wanted to free him from this pain and prognosis.

With my mind and heart aligned, my brain started processing the situation as if I were his medical provider and he were my patient (it was a knee story, after all). Only, I was thinking from the lens of physical therapy rather than surgery. As I heard him list off his extensive health history and the painful description of what he was experiencing, sympathy welled up in my heart for him. Aiden was in great pain, had undergone many surgeries, *and* had functional scoliosis — it was a lot to overcome.

Sitting there with my metaphorical medical cap on, I began thinking through all of Aiden's biomechanics that could be affected, the tissues that may be damaged, the weaknesses that would have to be strengthened, the compensation patterns that would have to be retrained, and the joints that would need to be realigned.

As I mentioned earlier in this book, my passion as an athletic trainer is the knee, hip, and lower extremity. I had a lot of ideas for non-surgical options, and just as important, since I now live as a Medical Intercessor and am aligned with God, I also had another partner to tap for help: God!

As Aiden shared his health history and decades-long journey leading to the pain he was experiencing, I accessed the many knowledge files and experiences I had stored within the left hemisphere of my brain. As I sat there, present and relaxed, listening to Aiden describe his symptoms and medical history, the left side of my brain sorted through all the knowledge files I had stored over the years; knowledge of the tissue and pathologies, knowledge of the biomechanics that were at stake, knowledge of the phenomenal modality advancements we now have to improve the health of the tissue, knowledge of physical therapy advancement, knowledge of the timelines needed to bring all of these together to make big improvements to the pain my friend was experiencing.

As I processed all of that knowledge, I started to come up with a treatment plan. It was a pretty lengthy protocol involving many modalities and specialists, and I started to come to the realization that Aiden may need to dedicate 18–24 months to various treatments and therapies. Although I believed he would improve drastically, I wasn't sure he could ever overcome his severe leg-length issue.

And then, as I considered all of this, my partner, God, dropped an image into the right hemisphere of my brain.

When God drops one of these images into my mind, I describe it as "a picture worth a thousand words" because the image comes with a lot of information that I just *know* to be true. In this particular mental image, I saw a man standing inside Aiden's lumbar spinal column. I *knew* the man standing in Aiden's spine was Aiden's adult son.

ALIGNMENT 6

My friendship with Aiden was fairly new, and I was unsure whether he even had an adult son. However, I *knew* that's what God had shown me. When I saw this image, I jumped back over to my left brain and recalled learning that chronic low back pain can be tied to carrying a spiritual load for a long time.

Without any certainty beyond the mental image in my mind that God had shared with me, I said, "Do you have an adult son who you have been carrying a load for? Maybe you have taken on a spiritual or emotional toll for him?"

Tears instantly formed in Aiden's eyes. He knew exactly what my vision meant.

"Yes," he finally managed to say. He then shared many, many years of emotional and spiritual pain he'd been carrying for a long time. Without a doubt, I knew this toilsome spiritual load was one of the contributing reasons for Aiden's nerve pain.

Aiden then shared that the son God showed me was his middle son from a previous marriage. He'd had zero communication with this son for more than 20 years. Aiden shared that he had two other children from the previous marriage, a younger daughter and an older son, both of whom also had strained relationships with him. Of the three, the daughter was the only one he'd had some contact with in the past few years. In addition to the physical issues related to his knee history, Aiden's heart and body were carrying the strain of these estranged relationships and an extraordinary amount of pain from the past, both of which were negatively impacting his health.

This is what divine knowing you can have access to when you partner with the God, the Great Physician, and co-labor with Him in your work. Through this partnership, I was able to see much more about Aiden's situation (spirit, mind, and body) than I would have had through my medical knowledge alone. God offers extraordinary solutions!

USING BOTH SIDES OF THE BRAIN

The approach I activated with Aiden that day was one of the techniques I teach more in depth in my courses. Be sure to find the ad in the back to learn how to become a ViaRayma Practitioner. We created the branded name, ViaRayma, because "via" means *the way*, the Greek word "rhema" (pronounced ray-ma) means *God's spoken word*, and "ray" symbolizes a *ray of hope* offered to the patient. Therefore, ViaRayma is the way to practice medicine partnered with God's spoken word, offering hope that supersedes science-based thinking.

This technique teaches you how to use both sides of your brain to be simultaneously present with your patient and with God. It's a unique experience. When I was sitting with my friend Aiden as he told me about his symptoms, I could actually feel the two sides of my brain processing simultaneously.

On the left side, my knowledge-and-expertise bank was thinking through all the options from a medical perspective. I knew we could get the nerve in a better position, improve blood flow to the nerve, improve the muscle function, or improve the alignment of the spine, pelvis, and all the soft tissues involved. Meanwhile, the right side of my brain was keeping me present as I listened to Aiden and waited for God to enter the conversation.

This ability to use both sides of your brain in the presence of your patient is what changes everything.

This ability to use both sides of your brain in the presence of your patient is what changes everything.

To begin practicing this technique, you need to find quiet time, prepare your mind, and let God speak to you — remember, "Be

ALIGNMENT 6

still and know God." This is also a time when you can speak to God. The technique requires two-way dialogue.

In Brian Heasley's book, *Be Still*, he describes the language "know God" as "*encounter Him*."[28] I like Brian's description of knowing God and interacting with God as an *encounter*. That's exactly what you feel: You encounter His presence rather than just *know* He exists.

This interaction only happens when you stop processing and thinking through all of the knowledge you have trained into your brain over many years to get to where you are. You have to pause that processing, be still, and allow God to move and give you something from Him for your patient.

Let's illustrate it this way. Take a look at Figure 8.2. The left hemisphere of your brain has stored many years of knowledge, skills, and experience and created a memory bank filled with resources to implement with every patient that comes to you. The right hemisphere is the creative and intuitive side of your brain that partners with God's divine wisdom and allows Him to drop something into your mind. You are called to store up knowledge and partner with God, and when you do so, it's like God is reaching into your memory bank and finding just the right knowledge file to implement with the perfect patient at the perfect time to bring perfect healing. Then God reaches into the memory bank of stored knowledge and grabs just the right solution for the next patient, and so on.

FIGURE 8.2 BRAIN HEMISPHERES SIMULTANEOUSLY WORKING WITH KNOWLEDGE AND DIVINE WISDOM PARTNERSHIP.

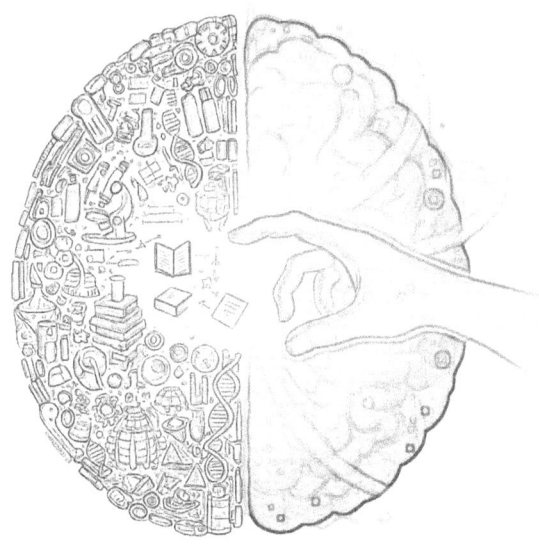

In the left hemisphere of your brain are the storehouses of knowledge, expertise, and skills you have developed throughout your experience. The right hemisphere, the brain's creative space, is the place where God's divine wisdom meets and partners with you, using your left-hemisphere knowledge and skills to their highest potential. It is this partnership that illustrates the work you do as a Medical Intercessor.

When your mind is aligned with your heart, your partnership with God works without any effort. When your mind veers away from your heart, it's hard to dig through and process all your stored knowledge for each and every patient. Partnering with God is the difference between an easy and light moment and an exhausting one.

Partnering with God is the difference between an easy and light moment and an exhausting one.

The alignment of your mind with your heart is done first through the alignment in God's love, in which your heart is renewed to God's heart. Then operating from your renewed mind (Spirit-led thinking) in alignment with your renewed heart, you walk in the power of God's love working through you. This doesn't only change your thinking; it changes your words.

WORDS HAVE POWER

The book of Proverbs is packed with wisdom. One of my favorite proverbs is "For as a man thinks in his heart, so is he" (Proverbs 23:7, NKJV).

When you invite Jesus to live in your heart, you can begin to align your soul with your Spirit and think with the mind of Christ. When you align your mind with this new heart, your thinking becomes flooded with the thoughts of God, followed by speaking from God.

Just as the proverb says, you will begin to speak differently because you are thinking differently — in your heart versus from your mind. Your words will naturally reflect this new approach.

This is a crucial shift because spoken words have power. God created the entire world by speaking words. He also taught us that speaking the name of Jesus is extremely powerful. Every one of the healing miracles performed by Jesus recorded in scripture happened because of His words. He spoke, and the dead lived again, the lame walked, the blind eyes opened, and the disease ended at the sound.

The same is true of the words you speak to your patients. You have the power to provide limited healing or true healing to those who seek your help simply by choosing to rely on your own knowledge alone or partnering with Him to use you as a

Medical Intercessor. Either your words will be limiting, or they will allow in His healing.

Our spoken words matter — partnership with heaven brings heaven!

God's will is that no disease, illness, injury, or infirmity prevail. The opposite of God's will is the will of the enemy, Satan. When you agree with a limited diagnosis or prognosis for a patient (even when it's very valid-seeming, based on all the in-depth knowledge you have gained from research, resources, and education), and you speak in that way to your patient, you're creating agreement with the enemy on behalf of your patient. However, if you are partnering with God as your Divine CEO and allow Him to work through you to heal your patient, you can use your words to invite true healing for your patient.

Up until this moment, you may never have thought about how the solutions you have to offer in the form of diagnosis and prognosis, while necessary paperwork within your profession, can be very limiting with regard to complete healing. Your written words have power too — your heart behind the written words dictates the negative or positive power.

THE DOUBLE RAINBOW DIAGNOSIS AND TREATMENT ARC

In scripture, the rainbow is a beautiful symbol of God's covenant with Noah; it is a promise never to destroy the earth by flood again. In patient treatment, the double rainbow is a symbol of hope for more than one treatment plan. Because we know that the tongue has the power of life and death (Proverbs 18:21, NIV), partnering with our Divine CEO to offer multiple solutions to our patients becomes a critical part of delivering true healing, according to His word.

A double rainbow forms when the refracted light that didn't exit the raindrop to form the primary rainbow reflects off the back of the raindrop again before exiting the drop, creating a second rainbow with inverted colors. It's even possible, though very rare, to have triple and quadruple rainbows. This can happen if enough light is held and reflected several times.[29]

FIGURE 8.3 DOUBLE RAINBOW

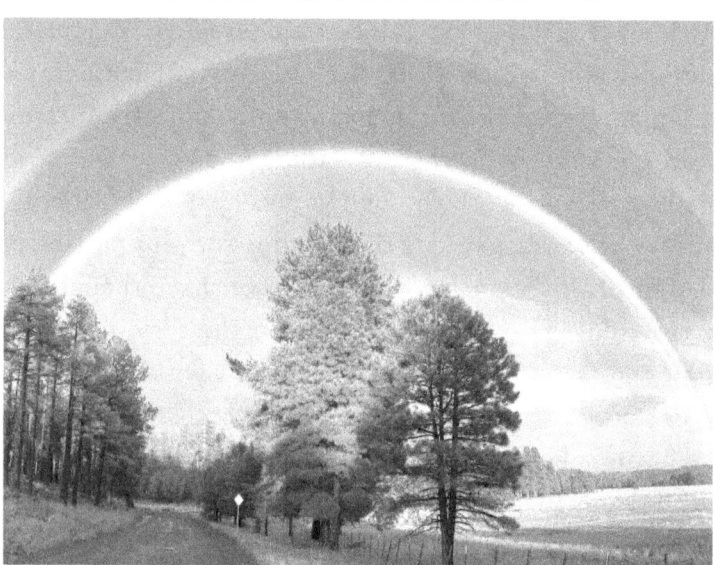

In patient treatment, this Double Rainbow diagnosis approach works as follows: Treatment happens in an arc, from Point A to Point B. When you interact with a patient and give them a diagnosis or assessment to identify what you are treating, you and your patient are standing at Point A. That assessment or diagnosis creates a pathway connecting to Point B, which is the solution for the patient's specific diagnosis or problem. Usually, Points A and B are science-based and identified according to your knowledge, expertise, and experience. In ViaRayma, we call this pathway from Point A to Point B the Primary Arc (equivalent to the primary rainbow).

But by now you know there is more hope to offer, so you provide an additional, parallel path for your patient — the secondary rainbow. This Secondary Arc also has a Point A and a Point B, but the Secondary Arc is formed from a divine ray of hope and the additional light left to release from the Primary Arc.

FIGURE 8.4 DOUBLE RAINBOW DIAGNOSIS

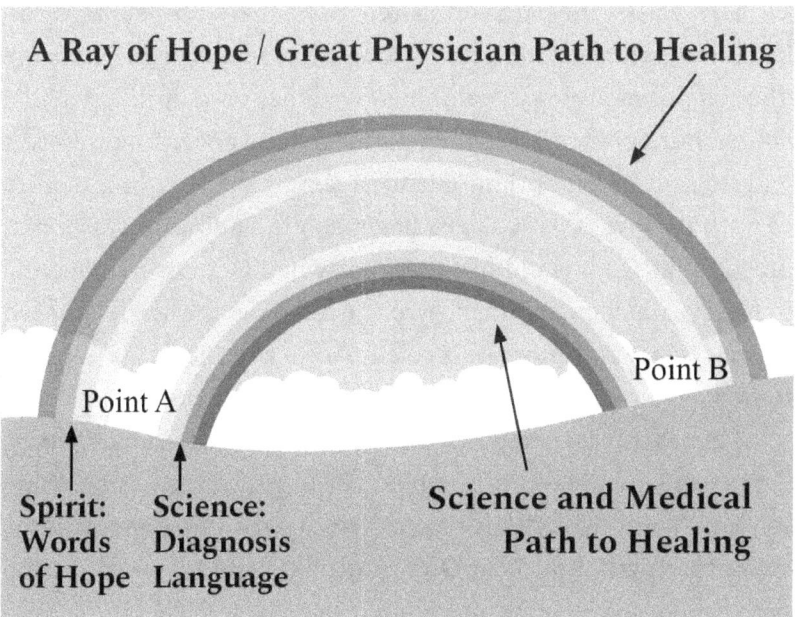

The Double Rainbow symbolizes the healing available through science and Spirit. Our medical knowledge gives us many options for our patients, symbolized by the Primary Arc. Meanwhile, God's divine wisdom brings another, second arc of healing that can eventually eliminate the need for the first arc entirely.

I find the double rainbow to be the perfect analogy. As illustrated in Figure 8.4, one pathway, the Primary Arc, is the science path, and the other pathway, the Secondary Arc, is the path of hope, light in the darkness, and faith as an alternative possibility. And just think, with enough light from the Holy Spirit, there could even be a third or fourth path connecting Point A to Point B!

ALIGNMENT 6

Do you recall the story I shared about my daughter, Deonna, who had seizures for nine years? Let's apply this double rainbow analogy to her diagnosis path.

One path the doctors gave her was from Point A (a diagnosis of epilepsy), through the arc of medicine and some dietary suggestions, and not much else, to Point B (fewer seizures). This plan only offered so much hope and definitely not complete healing.

That wasn't the path we desired for her. So we, as her faithful, believing parents with a background in some type of medicine (though not neurology), combined with her own faith, created a double rainbow for her, which allowed hope according to God's will, to still be an option. For nine years, we lived in a duality of both pathways as we gave her medicine and also spoke and prayed that God would heal her, but when God visited Deonna in her dream, her Secondary Arc canceled out the science-based Primary Arc, and she lives a seizure-free and medicine-free life to this day!

This is the same with the application for Aiden's story. One path was the out of the box, yet ingenious, solution using science. There would have definitely been some benefits if he chose that path. But then, God showed up and offered a second path, giving Aiden even more hope.

AIDEN'S DOUBLE RAINBOW DIAGNOSIS

Even in our first conversation, Aiden and I realized God was at work. However, His presence continued as Aiden followed the recommendations for physical healing.

Aiden had been in some pretty severe pain over the past two years, yet a short time after the first conversation, he told me that after only three weeks, he was 100 percent pain-free in his back and hip. During that time, he had been following his tissue-healing treatments and modalities, yet, he didn't credit his healing to only that.

Though his functional scoliosis was still present and no notable changes had occurred to the spinal column, hips, or knees, the combination of the Path of Spirit and the Path of Science had brought him not just a release from physical pain; it had also given him spiritual relief.

"Within twenty-four hours of the divine intervention, I was healed spiritually," he told me as we sat over a cup of coffee (one of our favorite meeting activities). "That night, God gave me a very vivid spiritual dream in which I got to see my son. I saw him freed from the captivity he has been living in through me, and I could see the presence of his love."

"And, not just that," he added, his eyes sparkling. "My other kids have started texting me."

Knowing those relationships had also been strained, I replied, "Oh, wow! When did this happen?"

"Not too long ago," he said. "Mother's Day, in fact." Only a couple weeks after God intervened.

I tried to remain quiet and listen while he spoke, but I was grinning from ear to ear. He saw my expression and he, too, smiled.

We both knew the tissue-healing methods and modalities would bring about amazing results, and the exercises he was doing were helpful, but nearly total healing in less than three weeks?

We knew the glory belonged to the Great Physician, the God of hope.

In a way, Aiden's entire situation is a perfect reflection of this new way of practicing medicine. His body was out of alignment, not just because of physical issues but because of spiritual ones he hadn't yet dealt with from some very painful relationships.

When I asked God for guidance in healing Aiden, I didn't know about Aiden's spiritual burdens, but God did. And simply by putting a question in my mind to ask my patient, God

ALIGNMENT 6

proceeded to start healing the other aspects in Aiden's life, not just his physical ailment. As He began to bring Aiden's physical body into alignment, He also began aligning Aiden's mind, emotions, and spirit in a way that would bring him more peace.

With his other relationships beginning to change for the better, he now has hope that the one with his still-estranged son will, too. There is a double rainbow in sight here for Aiden. And I believe wholeheartedly that God has this one in His hands! The Spirit of Joy and the Spirit of Peace have been released, and Aiden now operates with so much freedom!

This is what we can bring to our patients, with God's miraculous partnership. Let's not wait another day to start creating miracles. There are many, many more people like Aiden out there who need someone like you to enter their lives so that God can shower them with His blessings through you. And He already knows you are just the instrument to make it happen.

After all, that was exactly how He made you. It is my great hope that from now on, you will offer a double rainbow to all your patients and allow the light that still exists from God's promise to form a Secondary Arc with the delivery of a diagnosis or assessment. This secondary rainbow is the ray of hope that so many of our patients desperately need.

This hope is also what your heart desires — to be part of something greater than science alone. My heart, along with Aiden's, was healed by being part of this miracle. God wants that for you, too — and so do I.

THERE ARE MANY WAYS TO OFFER A RAY OF HOPE

As you can see, aligning your mind with your heart increases your power to help patients in unexpected ways — often exponentially. By realizing that your clinical knowledge can be a blessing or a roadblock, you can be more heart-centered and become aware when assumptions that result from your stored-up knowledge are getting in your way.

This balanced awareness will free you to tap more deeply into God's unified, expanded vision and to truly stand in the gap between God and your patient. When you are present in your mind, you live from your heart and let God lead. That's called Spirit-led medicine — when His Spirit of Wisdom is activated, and the eyes of your heart become enlightened (Ephesians 1:18, ESV). It allows you to make way for miracles.

With both small and large miracles in mind, think about different ways you can provide rays of hope. For instance, what if you have to inform a family that their three-year-old child has been diagnosed with a severe level of autism? There are a lot of programs and research studies that offer some improvements in these children over their lifespans, but typically, there is no ray of hope offered from the doctor's office. To give them one, you could encourage them that God is bigger than autism and that God offers healing for the impossible. You could invite them to seek hope through faith throughout this diagnosis journey.

I have observed this Double Rainbow treatment arc in my friends' life with their autistic daughter. Even though their daughter has not been completely healed from autism, she has had some pretty astounding breakthroughs that all the experts in her Primary Arc have no explanation for. My friends believe the Secondary Arc will eventually take over the science-based Primary Arc. That's a hope worth living for, even while living in a duality until then.

Here's another example. My son was diagnosed with a heart condition at a young age. The pediatric cardiologist we were referred to was a very kind-hearted soul and brought joy into the patient exam room, despite the difficult diagnosis.

That doctor encouraged us to work with our naturopathic doctor, who had a thought about what might be contributing to our son's heart disorder.

The naturopath ordered a series of blood and nutrient tests. From those results, she recognized that our son's enlarged heart was most likely caused by a nutrient absorption issue. Two years later, after following her instructions, my son's heart enlargement was resolved. That Secondary Arc — the ray of hope — changed the diagnosis and outcome for my son.

Imagine if we all started offering a ray of hope to every one of our patients.

We can do this by partnering not only with God, but with other specialties within the medical community and encouraging the patient to do so as well. I have a couple of friends who worked with a very knowledgeable naturopath during their Western medicine cancer treatments, and both of them had much better treatment results than their oncologist originally expected.

God works through others as well as through you, so I encourage you to get connected with others in the medical world who provide a service completely different from yours. You never know when God will use those connections to offer hope to your patient — and always leave room for miraculous recovery.

I partnered with God just the other day with one of my athletes whom I suspected had an observable Colles fracture. I splinted it and sent her to the emergency room for X-rays and a reset, but I also prayed that what I assessed with my own eyes was not the only option. I prayed and visualized both bones to align and for full healing to come into her.

Sure enough, the patient's parents texted me a few hours later stating that the physician said there was no fracture, and everything looked great. The patient didn't even have pain within a few hours after the injury. There was no natural way that what we experienced was a non-injury at the time I splinted the athlete due to swelling and deformity, but that Double Rainbow approach offered another way of healing from God as they transitioned from my care to the physician's care.

I could share story after story of positive patient outcomes that happen because of the conscious choice to partner with God, love deeply and intentionally, and invite encounters with Him to provide a ray of hope. These stories aren't just mine. So many people I've encountered since being commissioned by God to write this book have shared similar stories. Instead of including them all here (and making this book huge), I invite you to check out the ongoing testimonies that our community of ViaRayma practitioners create with this new way of practicing medicine. WhiteCoatRevival.com/testimony.

And most importantly, go and make your own double rainbows. Offer hope and healing to your patients!

When you do, be sure to share your stories with us as well.

ALIGNMENT 6

ALIGNMENT PAUSE

Reflection

1. Think about your interactions with your patients. How often do you find yourself present with them and really listening to them *without* processing your solution, your diagnosis, prognosis, or treatment plan? What can you change to be more still (Psalm 46:10)? The amount of time you get to spend with each patient is most likely the hardest thing to change. So, besides that factor, what can you do within yourself to be more present? What if you entered the treatment room with a still mind? What if you asked God to open your ears to hear something He wants you to hear, or to open your eyes to see something He wants you to see?

2. What do you think about the Double Rainbow diagnosis? Think about how you can offer a patient both the science behind their symptoms as well as the Great Physician's prognosis possibilities. Do you think this would be hard to implement? Practice being aware of your words with your next patient visit. It takes time to retrain your brain to ensure you offer both pathways to your patient.

3. What do you think about the possibility that something about your patient's disease, illness, injury, or infirmity may be tied to spiritual loads they are carrying? I encourage you to purchase *A More Excellent Way* by Dr. Henry W. Wright and use it as a reference for your patients when God leads you.

Activation

1. The ability to use both sides of your brain in the presence of your patient is something you can learn more about in the courses found in the ViaRayma community (see ad in back of book). You've chosen to align with love and to stand in the gap for your patient, so let's do a little practice right now.

   a. Practice using both sides of your brain simultaneously. In one of your next conversations, perhaps with a close friend or with a patient, practice the skill of listening to someone talk while simultaneously inviting God into the conversation.

   b. Ask God to show you something about that person and wait for the image that will come into your mind.

2. Read and reflect on Ephesians 1:18 (ESV): "The God of our Lord Jesus Christ, the Father of glory, may give you the Spirit of wisdom and of revelation in the knowledge of Him, *having the eyes of your hearts enlightened*, that you may know what is the hope to which He has called you."

3. Speak this decree: "Lord, open the eyes of my heart. I choose to lead with my renewed heart from this day forth. I receive Your Spirit of Wisdom activated within in me, choosing to partner with Your divine wisdom. Please forgive me. I repent from operating out of the Tree of the Knowledge of Good and Evil, and I no longer choose to lead from my knowledge alone. Lord, send me into the exam room as your vessel offering Double Rainbow Arcs —releasing hope and healing over every patient I encounter. I choose to think differently, speak differently, and practice differently, fully aligned with my transformed heart and mind."

ALIGNMENT 6

HOW IS THE BOOK RESONATING WITH YOU SO FAR?

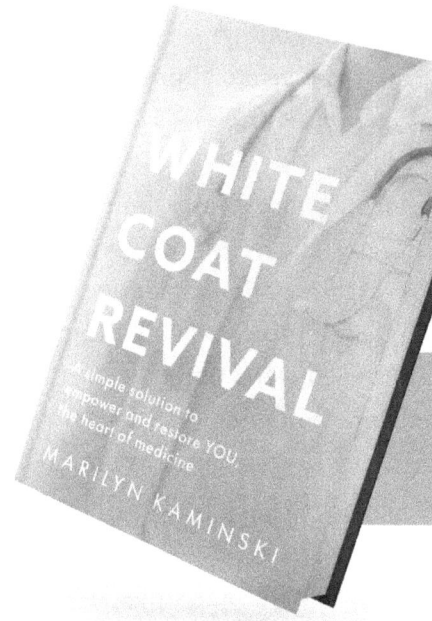

Have you felt the **immense power** it holds to transform the **medical world** as we know it?

Imagine the ripple effect this knowledge could create!

Help others discover this GAME-CHANGING book by leaving a review.

Your words can ignite A POWERFUL MOVEMENT!

WhiteCoatRevival.com/Book-Review

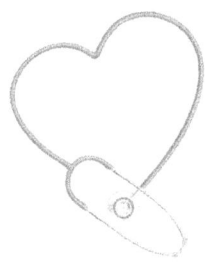

Chapter 9

ALIGNMENT 7: ALIGN SCIENCE WITH SPIRIT – PARTNER WITH HEAVEN

We are co-workers with God and you are
God's cultivated garden, the house he is building.

— 1 CORINTHIANS 3:9 (TPT)

Wisdom comes from those who have understanding (Proverbs 10:12, NKJV). Alignment 7 happens when you understand God's full plan for the healing and your very essential role you play in the finished work of His plan. He created you on purpose ***to find His hidden treasures***: to gain extraordinary knowledge of His handiwork and use science-based evidence of His prize creation, the human body, ***so that you would then partner with Him and co-labor with Him and your stored knowledge to heal!*** (Psalm 19 and Proverbs 8:12, NKJV)

ALIGNMENT 7

It is my goal that you do not close this book without gaining this understanding. That partnership is the Spirit component of this Alignment. When you understand that God's original design was for science and Spirit to work in unity, God will begin to show off *through* you!

This capstone step is about seeking and embodying the partnership with God's omniscient wisdom so that your decisions, interventions, and presence as a Medical Intercessor reflect a perfect balance between knowledge and eternal truth. Remember, God created you on purpose for a purpose and for His promises to be fulfilled here on earth. Therefore, you, the one who holds a lot of science-based knowledge and expertise about the human body, are equally as important to the mission of delivering true healing as the presence of God's Holy Spirit. The combination of the two is the solution that balances the constantly swinging pendulum between the different approaches to medicine. This balanced approach doesn't allow either Spirit or science to be more important than the other. Instead, the pendulum becomes balanced and still as we use practical knowledge from both sides.

> *You, the one who holds a lot of science-based knowledge and expertise about the human body, are equally as important to the mission of delivering true healing as the presence of God's Holy Spirit. The combination of the two is the solution that balances the constantly swinging pendulum between the different approaches.*

With that in mind, in this chapter you'll gain a deeper understanding of the value of both approaches and how to unify them.

One thing I noticed with almost every vision I received was that God was illustrating two sides — one science and one Spirit. As I came to know the full message He was sending, it became very clear that **science without Spirit and Spirit without science**

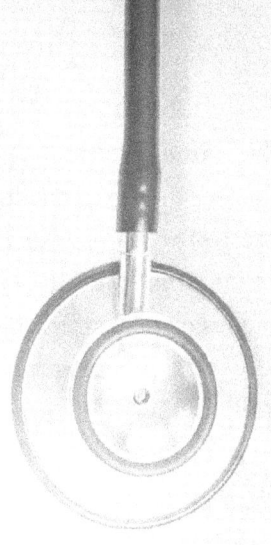

Science without Spirit and Spirit without science are the same problem: Each is only half of the equation.

are the same problem: Each is only half of the equation. Whether it's on a large scale with a pendulum swinging from one extreme to the other over many thousands of years, or a small, individual situation with a person gravitating between the two approaches or pedestals, the problem remains the same.

God's design was never meant for us to research, study, and apply our knowledge alone. He always intended for us to store that extraordinary knowledge in our minds and use it as we partner with His mind for action.

This new approach I present to you recognizes that science is the knowledge of the physical world through observable facts and events while also acknowledging God's divine orchestration throughout the physical world. Therefore, understanding the necessity of integrating the power of the Holy Spirit is essential to fulfilling your purpose to fulfill God's will according to His promise.

The previous six alignments and each of the visions I shared with you had both a spirit component and a science component. See Figure 9.1. All along, God intended for the co-laboring of both. Are you ready to bring medicine back to God's original design?

FIGURE 9.1 SUMMARY OF ALIGNMENTS AND ILLUSTRATIONS THROUGHOUT THIS BOOK

ALIGNMENTS	SCIENCE	SPIRIT
Alignment #1: God's Vision	Man's Vision	God's Vision
Alignment #2: Purpose	Path of Soul - Vocation in Medicine	Path of Spirit - God's Plan for Your Purpose
Alignment #3: Soul & Spirit	Soul	Spirit
Alignment #4: Hope Expectations	Wishful Thinking for Healing	Confident Expectation for Healing
Alignment #5: Love	Situational	Stand in the Gap
Alignment #6: Mind & Heart	Lead from Mind and Leave Heart Behind	Lead from Your Heart's Desire
Alignment #7: Science & Spirit	Science - Human Knowledge	Spirit - God's Omniscience
ILLUSTRATIONS	SCIENCE	SPIRIT
Pedestal Leaders Illustration	Path of Science	Path of Spirit
Overswung Pendulum Illustration	Western Approach	Eastern Approach
Purpose Alignment Arc	Seeking Desired Knowledge	Seeking Relationship with God
Thinking Ways	Soul-led Thinking	Spirit-led Thinking
Wisdom Pyramid	Knowledge and Data	Divine Wisdom
Brain Hemispheres	Knowledge Processing	Divine Wisdom
Double Rainbow	Primary Arc - Science and Medical Language	Secondary Arc - Spirit and Spoken Words of Hope

GOD'S OMNISCIENT WISDOM IS HERE FOR US

Due to the current medical system's chains and boundaries, we must maneuver around and through many obstacles that stand in our way when we treat our patients. Sometimes our expertise and amazing knowledge get halted by rules, regulations, insurance hurdles, pharmaceutical strongholds, corporate greed, and more. When these halted moments occur, God can meet us with divine wisdom.

His divine wisdom always soars over these obstacles. He is God. He will not give us divine wisdom that does not take into account the law of the land. Only solutions we devise for our patients without His partnership are limited by these obstacles. When our human brain cannot process the solution, we can tap into the omniscient mind of Christ, and His ways are greater than ours (Isaiah 55:8–9, NKJV). Because of this, miraculous solutions sometimes pop into our minds from Him. They often appear so simple that we cannot believe we didn't think of the solution on our own.

The Apostle Paul explains to us throughout his letter to the people of Ephesus how we access God's omniscient wisdom. When Jesus died and rose again, God sent the Holy Spirit here on earth for us to access and partner with Him through the power of the Holy Spirit (Ephesians 2:18, NLT). We can receive God's wisdom through the power of the Holy Spirit communicating to us in our spirit through intuition or discernment. God will speak to us through scripture (the Living Word). Also, we receive wisdom when we ask Him and tune in to hear His still, small voice through words. Sometimes we receive His answers in pictures "worth a thousand words," or that have a divine weight to them.

When I was receiving daily visions, dreams, and downloads from God about this new approach to medicine and the reason for writing this book, I had less knowledge of what the Bible had to say specifically about God's will for healing. But every day, I would ask God for His direction. I would sit with my Bible and thumb through the pages until I believed God was stopping me and telling me to read there. These are still some of my favorite moments of seeking His wisdom. I am floored by the number of passages that were absolutely perfect answers to my prayer to God when I'd say, "Help me understand what you are showing me."

One of the first passages God showed me was something I had read thousands of times throughout my life, but that day, I saw words jumping off the page that I had not really thought about before: "Your will be done on earth as it is in heaven" (Matthew 6:10, NKJV). This would happen time and time again. I located Bible verses I didn't even know existed. I was not a Bible college student or anything even close to it. I didn't attend a Christian primary or secondary school where I was required to memorize and be tested on Bible verses like my kids are, but I believed I knew a lot of the contents inside the Bible due to the number of church sermons I'd heard and Bible study groups I'd participated in over the years.

Because I asked God for answers and was set to open the Bible to learn something new, He was able to speak to me straight through the Bible passages. As I was learning these new passages, I desired more — more wisdom and more wisdom. I wanted to know more. Learn more. Understand more.

I wrote this book for you so you could also receive His amazing wisdom. As you now know since you have read this far, God has an extraordinary plan for you to do even more for the advancement of His Kingdom and to serve your patients with even greater love. The first step is for you to learn what's possible.

Here are two passages that stood out to me regarding what is possible:

1. "Your will be *done on earth as it is in heaven*" (Matthew 6:10, NKJV).
2. "Most assuredly, I say to you, he who believes in me, the works that I do he will do also; and *greater works than these he* will do, because I go to My Father" (John 14:12, NKJV).

On earth? Wait. *On earth*. That means we don't have to wait until we get to heaven for healing. Do greater works than Jesus? Whoa! Jesus's adult life on earth was filled with healing miracles. Can we do more?

These two verses greatly expanded my understanding about what's possible with healing.

YOUR KNOWLEDGE + HIS OMNISCIENCE = MORE POTENTIAL

When I unpacked God's full message to me, for you, I knew the solution for your well-being and the medical system would be solved by the alignment of science and Spirit. I call it *Holy Spirit Medicine* in which intercessors who are medically trained are interceding for the patient to bring heaven here on earth. With this powerful relationship — two-way communication with an omniscient (all-knowing) partner — **you should never have to guess what's wrong with a patient again. You should never need to agree to a diagnosis or a prognosis as final say ever again. Anything is possible with God!** He will meet your mind with His mind and reveal the

You should never have to guess what's wrong with a patient again.

answers to you through the power of the Holy Spirit and the Mind of Christ — all *within* you and your mind!

With that in mind, despite our Divine CEO's magnificent power, inviting His wisdom in to assist you is only half of the partnership. You also will want to seek to increase your own wisdom because the only limit to what you can do with God comes from within.

The only limit to what you can do with God comes from within.

To explain, let's revisit my friend Aiden's story from the previous chapter. When he ran through his history with me and communicated to me what he desired as the outcome, I started thinking of all the medical advancements we now have available for tissue health and the supercool therapy exercises, modalities, and techniques I have stored in my knowledge to remedy his problem.

My extensive knowledge in this area could have offered quite a bit of hope to Aiden without the divine wisdom God dropped in. However, God prompted me to bounce back into my knowledge files within the left side of my brain and access something else — something I wouldn't have thought of on my own. With the vision He gave me, I recalled that sometimes when people have chronic low back problems, it can mean they are carrying a heavy load in the spirit.

God could use this information to guide me because I had expanded my knowledge — my convergence point with God's Divine Wisdom — to at least be aware of the teachings of authors like Henry Wright, writer of *The More Excellent Way*, who took the time to learn and teach others about this magnificent information. Through that awareness, God was able to nudge me to ask Aiden if he felt that he was carrying a heavy load for his son.

If I had not been aligned and partnering with God, and if I had not had that bit of extra awareness, I might have stuck to just working with Aiden to see how he could take power over his injury through strength training, physical therapy, and many tissue-healing modalities and nutrients. And yet, that wouldn't have been enough. Instead, since I had that extra bit of awareness and was able to receive God's omniscient wisdom to use it for my friend that day, I could offer a ray of hope in addition to the scientific and medical path to the outcome he was desiring for his back pain. And I have been filled with joy as I've watched Aiden make huge strides in recovering from his back pain, avoid another surgery, and live a life free from a burden he was silently carrying!

Increasing your opportunities for partnership with Him isn't about how much knowledge you have in one area, but about becoming knowledgeable in many areas.

The more knowledge you store, even simple awareness of other modalities of healing, the more opportunities He has to meet you with His divine wisdom. Increasing your opportunities for partnership with Him isn't about *how much* knowledge you have in one area, but about becoming knowledgeable in many areas.

When we step out of our specialty lane within our profession and expand our knowledge in other areas of health and medicine, we become more aware of what's possible. Our possibilities expand, and we become open to different convergence opportunities met by God. What you have learned in this book has already exponentially expanded what's possible when you stand in authority wearing the white coat!

When we have more knowledge, God has more opportunities to show us different paths toward healing and meet us where we are so we can understand His vision. Please don't mistake that for gaining more knowledge *and then processing it all on your own*, which would defeat the whole point of this book.

With Aiden's situation, God was only able to share a spiritual component contributing to Aiden's back and hip pain because I had expanded my knowledge with regard to spiritual ties being potential reasons for physiological symptoms. If I had not been aware of that possibility, God would not have been able to meet Aiden that day through me. There would not have been a convergence point for divine wisdom to meet my stored-up knowledge.

When you are gaining knowledge, it's as if you're getting training that brings you up a level or two in your ability to understand God's language. This is something that can surely help your patients as you can effectively work to bring what God is showing you into fruition, sometimes in unexpected ways.

BE A WISE PARTNER

God's wisdom can do the impossible, but He will only go where He is invited. He gives us the free will, in our own timing, to come to Him. Because of this, we must also be wise about how the enemy works. Mainly, the enemy uses lies to fool us into believing we have no power or there's no hope, and the impossible and unexplainable creates a stop wall.

Fortunately, all you have to do to triumph over the enemy is to expand your knowledge of God, love Him, surrender to Him, and be grateful He called you to be the vessel for Him to carry hope and healing. All you have to do is believe it. It is done. It is written. It is finished. It's available to all who believe. It's always been there. Just believe it, activate it, and live it out. And close your ears to all those who will tell you miraculous healings are not possible. This book will create a new way of thinking for sure, but

This book will create a new way of thinking.

beware of all those who will strip your excitement for these new possibilities. The enemy is sly. Measure everything against the Living Word, not against the opinions of others.

What lies from the enemy have you been living with? What wrong teachings have entered your mind and taken up residency when they shouldn't have? What understanding is being blocked?

I have been coaching and mentoring allopathically trained medical physicians in the Western medical system for a couple of years now, and I'm struck by the number of lies they've accepted from the leaders they trusted. So many have been taught to shun spiritual methods and even some natural healing, such as nutrition and herbal remedies. They completely distrust these and steer clear of integrating either solution into their practice despite evidence that they work. In fact, they fear practicing their own spirituality at all in their daily work. These fears are the result of the direct actions of the enemy at work in the form of limited education or lies.

All of these wrong teachings must be undone. Wrong teachings can prevent you from hearing and receiving truth. You will need to learn to recognize the lies and recode your mind with truth that only comes from above. Be sure to download the supplemental content (see the ad in the back of the book). I have some guided audios to help you reveal lies and replace them with truths. This sanctification process is necessary to be the Medical Intercessor God called you to be.

Seek wisdom. Read your Bible daily. Spend time in two-way conversation with God. Turn away from the wicked. Study truth. There are more than 200 Bible verses listed in this book. Study them. Pair up with a mentor or a coach to navigate this amazing wisdom.

Ephesians 6:13 (NKJV) instructs us to "take up the whole armor of God, that you may be able to withstand in the evil day, and having done all, to stand." The whole Armor of God consists of the belt of truth, the breastplate of righteousness, the boots of the gospel, the shield of faith, the helmet of salvation, and the sword of the Spirit as the Living Word of God.

All of these are important, but the one I find to be most important is the sword. We can sharpen our double-edged sword by staying in God's Living Word. When you have Bible verses turning in your mind all day, your mind is protected from the enemy, and you can bring the presence of Christ into your day-to-day work more simply.

Study the life of Jesus. Study the Gospels. The Gospels share with us that God sent Jesus to live as a human so we can better relate and understand who God is and what is possible with Him. I love using the book *Quest 52* and *The Chosen* video series as ways to illustrate the love, power, and possibilities of what God can do through us when we choose to be a vessel for Him here on earth.[30] Expand your knowledge of how much the impossible and the unexplainable can be made reality if we partner with Him.

When our minds fill up with doubt, pride, or greed, or we limit our capabilities by relying only on our limited knowledge, then the enemy can prevent Christ from working through us. However, when we make it a habit to read from the Bible each day, sharpening our swords and understanding what's possible with God, our minds can receive all that God has for us. God will highlight certain words on the pages and download an unexplainable understanding as you read His word. It is unlike any other book you'll read, including this one.

Seek More Miracles

Let's go back to the importance of seeking knowledge of miracles we explored in Alignment 4. This is a transformative step. When you realize you are missing something and you seek for and find the answers you need, the truth can be liberating.

Prior to 2024, I did not know just how often someone could experience miraculous healings. I believed it was maybe a once-in-a-lifetime experience if you won the miracle lottery.

Even despite personally experiencing a miraculous healing of my appendix in 2021, I still didn't seek out more stories like what I'd experienced prior to my awakening in 2024. I was blind to the possibility of more complete healings because I was not looking for them. I was not seeking. God says if we seek, we shall find (Matthew 7:7 NKJV). When you seek to know about miracles, you'll learn about them. And when you seek to help create them, they will manifest.

When you seek to know about miracles, you'll learn about them. And when you seek to help create them, they will manifest.

What changed? The only difference between past me and present me is that *I started seeking to expand my knowledge in this area.*

I began by studying John G. Lake's books, who he was, and how he documented many thousands of miraculous healings. I read F.F. Bosworth's book, *Christ the Healer.*[31] Then I was exposed to Andrew Wommack and read his book, *God Wants You Well.*[32] Then someone invited me to a Global Celebrations week-long online forum.[33] The forum was phenomenal because there were people from all parts of the world teaching and sharing how healing miracle after healing miracle flowed through them as they stood in the gap and became vessels for God.

I encourage you to review the list of resources I have provided within the free 7 Alignments Supplemental Content to help you begin expanding your knowledge and exposing yourself to the vast number of miracles happening every day. And don't stop there. Please seek your own sources as well.

I also encourage you to listen to authors and speakers in person, meet them in person, and find a mentor to walk you

ALIGNMENT 7

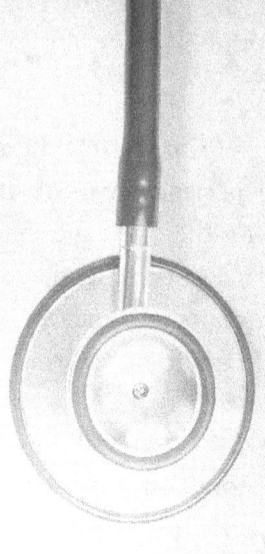

Your commitment to excellence and His commitment to loving you release a power this world has never seen before!

through and unpack all this newly gained knowledge. If you desire coaching and mentorship with me, I would love to walk through this journey with you. Check out the ad at the back of this book for more information.

Medicine was always meant to have a balance of the Holy Spirit and science. God chose you to bring both of those elements into the care you deliver to all your patients. He equipped you to walk in your purpose and your power, exercising the authority He has called you to as one who balances your extraordinary knowledge with God's omniscient wisdom to heal your patient.

Your commitment to excellence and His commitment to loving you release a power this world has never seen before! The pursuit you have always longed for, to be aligned with God at work, not just out of work, is possible.

ALIGNMENT

7

ALIGNMENT PAUSE

Reflection

1. What are you feeling after reading this book so far? Do you feel encouraged to integrate your faith into medicine — the Medical Intercessor/Holy Spirit-led way? Do you feel hopeful to witness complete healings or even miracles?

2. Integrating one's faith into medicine has been an uphill battle for decades. What do you think about the integration of your faith the way it is presented in this book — simply by co-laboring with God in your thoughts and operating from the mind of Christ? Please understand this integration is all within you! It's *you* aligning heart and mind, soul and spirit, within you. Your patient may have no idea that you are operating with your mind under the influence of God's amazing power. This is a way to integrate faith within your work. This is different than an evangelistic approach. Both approaches can be used if God leads you and the patient receives, but I encourage you to ask God which approach He wants you to implement and not assume praying is the only way to bring the presence of Christ into the room.

3. In your next patient interaction, take a moment and pause from the diagnosis, prognosis, or treatment plan you will implement. Ask God to partner with you while you are interacting with the patient. The patient doesn't need to know you are partnering with Him at that moment. Stand present in front of your patient with an abundance of stored knowledge in your mind, but silently, within your mind, ask God what He wants to show you. Be still and wait a few seconds. Did something come

to mind that you would not have thought of at that moment? Did a solution present itself that you didn't think of before — different than what the left hemisphere of your brain was thinking?

a. Don't discount the thought, even if your own understanding cannot comprehend. Ask God again if there is anything else He wants to show you. When you first are practicing, it's okay not to move with confidence. Hold onto the thought. Write it down. You can always revisit it later to confirm until you gain more confidence of knowing what is God's voice and what is not.

b. If you did move forward with what God showed you, keep record of it so you can do your own little case study as you are practicing. Did the treatment go substantially better than you thought was possible? Did you notice the patient was more peaceful than expected? Did you discover a deeper underlying problem that you or the patient may not have been aware of without God's partnership?

Activation

1. Read and reflect on John 14:26 (NKJV): Jesus said, "The Helper, the Holy Spirit, whom the Father will send in My name, He will teach you all things and bring to your remembrance all things that I have said to you."

2. Speak this decree: "I use my knowledge and talents according to Matthew 25 to further God's will here, on earth. I acknowledge God as my source for calling, wisdom, and strength. I do not discount the natural wisdom I have gained, and I invite God's divine wisdom to illuminate what is needed in every patient interaction. I

ALIGNMENT

7

expect to follow God and partner with Him for healing, more and more!"

3. Revisit John 14:12 (NKJV). I have mentioned this verse multiple times throughout this book. Recite this passage often. Jesus says, "Most assuredly, I say to you, he who believes in Me, the works that I do **he will do also**; and **greater works than these he will do**, because I go to My Father." Do you now know why Jesus said, "*greater works than these*"? You have the ability to partner your expertise and medical knowledge *with* God through the power of His Holy Spirit. When Jesus performed miracles, He did not have medical knowledge. His skill was in the trade of carpentry, not medicine. How much more are you equipped than even Jesus was? I find that to be one of the most fascinating revelations God has given me to share with you. Be empowered!

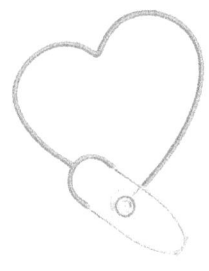

Chapter 10

THE NEW WAY: ALIGNED AND PARTNERED WITH GOD

And we know that all things work together for the good to those who love God, to those who are the called according to His purpose.

— ROMANS 8:28 (NKJV)

Congratulations on working through this transformation process to living in 100 percent alignment with God. Now that you've come through the 7 Alignments and your own misalignments are healed, you are truly equipped to go forth and heal others!

I'm excited to meet you someday and hear your transformation story. Be sure to journal about all changes you experience, even small ones. Journaling and speaking about your transformation journey are extremely powerful.

You will probably not be surprised to hear that this transformation will likely affect you in far greater ways than just in your vocation. After all, God sees you as a whole person with a life beyond your profession. Prepare for other transformations beyond your work in your career too. Living 100 percent aligned with God is your new way of life — vocation and personal life as one with Him. That's God's way.

Now that you've partnered with God as a co-creator for your life, the maze of seeming complexities and complications will begin to fall away, allowing a whole new future to unfold for you. Let's close out with a glimpse of what that future looks like. We'll look at what this transformation really means, and how you can move forward with the new knowledge and approach you've been empowered with from this book.

YOU HAVE POWER AS GOD'S CHOSEN PARTNER

You, as a Medical Intercessor, believe in the Almighty God *and* have a lot of knowledge of God's prize creation, the human body. You have skills and expertise that have taken years, maybe even decades, to obtain. Those years of experience and the expertise you have are a huge and necessary blessing! God will eagerly put them to use in this new way, now that you are fully aligned with Him.

Just as God chose you as His partner in healing, your patients also chose you to be the authority to give them solutions to their problem. When they scheduled an appointment with you and entered your exam room, they gave you permission to be the authority on the problem they presented to you. With that authority, you can now offer two solutions: one based on your left brain, and one based on your intuitive, God-connected right brain.

I don't know of any patient who would say, "Doctor, please only give me one option. Please do not give me all of your knowledge and all of your hope and all of your solutions." They came to you for all of your knowledge, including your knowledge of who God is. You can give them the Double Rainbow diagnosis, which allows for countless possibilities sourced only from the God of all hope.

And remember, because it is not all up to you, the burden is lifted. You are not called to be the savior or the Messiah; you are only called to believe in Him and be sowers of His love. Let the Great Physician partner with you and watch what happens to patient outcomes. Expect many stories of miracles to appear. This has certainly been my experience, and we know that God shows no favoritism (Galatians 2:6, NIV). Why should He not give you the same kind of experience?

Let the Great Physician partner with you and watch what happens to patient outcomes. Expect many stories of miracles to appear.

It's Time to Claim Your Inheritance

I read a great analogy describing the understanding that God's grace has already been given to us.[34] Think about a situation where a banker calls you and tells you that you have an inheritance sitting in the bank. It's been sitting here for a while, but they haven't been able to get a hold of you. They inform you it's all yours, no strings attached, but you have to come down to the bank and get it. They cannot give it to anyone else, and they cannot change it over into your name unless you come down to claim it.

If you never come get it, it's still yours, but there is no value transferred to you. If you come down and claim it, then the large inheritance will be available in your account. All you have to do is come and get it. It's free. It's been given to you. You just have to take formal ownership of it.

This scenario is the same thing when it comes to accepting God's promise for you. He has already given it to you. It's free. You just have to choose to claim it. **Choose to claim this promise on your life and activate your God-given purpose!**

Mark 11:24 (ESV) says, "Therefore I tell you, whatever you ask in prayer, *believe that you have received it*, and *it* will be yours." **If you can see it, you can have it!** If you want your patients to experience miracle healings, start meditating on your patients being healed as you stand in the gap and flow the love of Christ and your patients will be healed right before your very eyes!

God has predestined and chosen you (Ephesians 1:11, NKJV). Each one of us has a purpose to fulfill for His will to be done here on earth (Philippians 2:13, NIV). You get to live your own story, and no one can know the full story of what God is doing in your life. However, I know God has prepared good works for you to do and that your stories are part of a larger, ongoing narrative. This alignment with His promise will transform many lives through your role within the medical world.

> *I know God has prepared good works for you to do and that your stories are part of a larger, ongoing narrative. This alignment with His promise will transform many lives through your role within the medical world.*

You are not leaving this book empty-handed. You now carry a new lens, a new authority, and a more purpose-filled assignment. Go forward as a Medical Intercessor who is not perfect, but who is aligned, equipped, and never alone.

I am here for you. I am already praying for you.

"May the Lord bless you and keep you; May the Lord make His face shine upon you, and be gracious to you; The Lord lift up His countenance upon you, and give you peace" (Numbers 6:24–26, NKJV).

YOU ARE A VESSEL FOR POURING OUT GOD'S LOVE

Just as you are not meant to be hopeless, you are also not meant to live a divided life. In your family, marriage, society, health, and profession, wherever you are, you're still the same person.

Living in alignment with God will stop the feeling of living trapped internally with a double mindset or a disconnect between your heart's desire and your mind's training that keeps you from being your true, authentic self. Instead, you can now live aligned with Christ and be authentic everywhere you go. That alignment will make you one with your purpose and God's will for you.

Mother Theresa once said, "I'm a little pencil in the hand of a writing God, who is sending a love letter to the world."[35] We are all called to be exactly that, a vessel or instrument spreading God's abundant love.

Dr. Elizabeth Vaughan, a world-renowned eye surgeon, says she is "an instrument in God's hand."[36] I love this. Be His instrument. Don't try to live life with your own power; it's exhausting and overwhelming. The instrument does nothing without the operator. The operator of the instrument does everything. Let God be your operator. His power is infinitely greater than yours. I urge you to align with God, partner with Him, and display His mighty workmanship in your daily work as a white coat and be the ray of light that forms the beautiful double rainbow for each and every patient!

Dr. Ben Carson is known for several surgeries widely regarded as miraculous. He believed that God was the divine orchestrator — sending patients to him and sending him to perform operations others deemed impossible. This conviction enabled him to enter the operating room with a confidence rooted not in himself but in submission to God. As Dr. Carson once prayed,

"Lord, from now on, you be the neurosurgeon, and I'll be the hands."[37] What might happen if we all adopted that posture? God calls us to pursue expertise and knowledge diligently, but then to yield — allowing Him to work through us as His vessels.

We are called to be God's vessels — both in the sense of a ship that carries treasures and in the sense of the vessels within the body that carry life itself. A vessel does not act on its own; it is directed by the hand of the operator. Likewise, blood vessels do not generate life; they carry the lifeblood where it is needed. In the same way, God works through us, partnering with the knowledge and expertise we hold. Our purpose is to assist the Great Physician, allowing His divine wisdom and healing love to flow through us as naturally as blood flows through the body — reaching the ends of the earth, one patient at a time.

A couple of months after I started writing this book, a friend sent me this prophetic note:[38]

> God is raising up Medical Intercessors with in-detail, intuitive understanding of the human body and its intricate processes. The unlocking of their calling and heart to heal will equip and release them to pray specifically targeted prayers into the inner workings of the human body to release greater levels of healing in the body of Christ, both in and outside of the church building. This strategic level of prayer-focused healing has not yet been released because many of these medical practitioners have channeled and directed their practical wisdom and knowledge toward pharmaceuticals, medical tests, and healing through traditional medical avenues.
>
> I see highly trained doctors and medical professionals praying over patients with such a

high level of diagnostic understanding and seeing body functions change as a result of these prayers. A lid needs to be lifted off their expertise so that it can be used to unlock very specific healing mechanisms within the human body as they pray prayers of faith and target specific body systems and functions with the healing power of Christ. Their prayers will be laser-focused down to the cellular and micro-function level.

I see that this will operate both in church prayer, intercession, and healing teams as well as in medical offices and hospitals across the world. God will equip them with such pinpointed, visual prayers that it will be as if they are looking at an MRI or other medical imaging and praying with such targeted vision, in the spirit, to see those results literally shift and move in the spiritual realm, but this will be expressed in the physical expression of amazing healings.

They also need to be empowered to bring these supernatural prayer frameworks into their areas of work, and they will start to see medical documentation that supports and affirms the miracles they are praying into. The enemy has resisted a Holy Spirit environment that combines the power of medical knowledge with the faith atmosphere of healing. God wants to start to shift this for His Kingdom to come into the scientific and medical world.

The words of her Spirit-filled prayer message are very profound and will no doubt transform you from a wishful thinker into a declarer of healing with confident expectation, according to God's will. I encourage you to speak this into your life.

Let's free ourselves from burden and take on the easy and light yoke that comes when we choose to be one with Christ everywhere we go.

STEP INTO A FUTURE OF PEACE AND JOY

Recall the vision I described in Chapter 3, in which the white coat was sitting in a fog with chains holding them down, helpless, and only able to offer their patient limited hope.

The happy news is that you are not called to be chained and only offer hopelessness. When you align with God and live out your God-given purpose, you are partnered with the God of hope (Romans 15:13, NKJV), and His will and His promise are fulfilled here on earth as in heaven. You are called to heal God's children, your patients.

You are not limited to what you alone, without Christ, have to offer. You have the science-based diagnosis, prognosis, and treatment pathway to direct your patient on, which is a form of hope, but you are also called as a child of God to offer greater hope and complete healing. You can be a vessel of this amazing healing because you now have a mind that takes on the mind of Christ.

Choosing to align your heart's desire and your mind is what broke you out of the chains of misalignment and dual mindsets. His ways are higher than our ways (Isaiah 55:9, NKJV). Created by deception, those chains will continue to exist for those who allow themselves to be bound by them.

You don't have to be chained and limited. You have the power and choice to free yourself. What would the world look like if more white coats took that unchained path?

Throughout the time while I was writing this book, God continued to show me visions of hospital lights turning off because the rooms held no patients, while instead, playgrounds filled with laughter. He showed me white coats with smiles growing bigger, hearts radiating a brighter red color, and white coats shining more brightly.

He showed me white coats rising above the fog and circling the whole earth, all with large, bright smiles, bright hearts, and chains and fog completely vanishing. He showed me how the patients would interact with the white coats and how they would walk away filled with joy, hope, peace, and healing.

This can be you as you join the *White Coat Revival.*

Preparing your mind and inviting divine wisdom from the Great Physician to partner with you for each patient interaction, and allowing the power of Christ to flow through you, will bring more healing than our traditional prayers alone.

This book is here to create a mindset change, not an evangelistic approach to healing. Simply by inviting Christ into your day and being one with Him in your mind, you bring His presence to your patients. Praying with your patients when that amazing opportunity arises is great and is strongly encouraged. But preparing your mind and inviting divine wisdom from the Great Physician to partner with you for each patient interaction, and allowing the power of Christ to flow through you, will bring more healing than our traditional prayers alone.

In 2 Peter 1:2–4 (NKJV), Simon Peter declares for us, "Grace and peace be multiplied to you in the knowledge of God and of Jesus our Lord, as His divine power has given to us all things that pertain to life and godliness, through the knowledge of Him who called us by glory and virtue, by which have been given to us exceedingly great and precious promises, that **through these you may be partakers of the divine nature,** having escaped the corruption that is in the world."

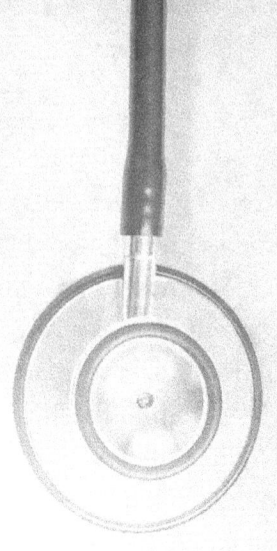

When you choose to partner with God, miracles will flow from your fingertips. You will be the vessel He has called you to be — one who will bring healing as great as the works Jesus did here on earth.

When you choose to partner with God, miracles will flow from your fingertips. You will be the vessel He has called you to be — one who will bring healing as great as the works Jesus did here on earth.

This mindset shift is a combination of *Who* you work with — God, as your CEO — and *how* you work with Him. This *how* is important because you must remember that His vision and His way are different from those of any other CEO. He has a different idea of integrating faith into our science-based profession. He is the balance we need in all aspects of our lives, including but not limited to our careers. Are you ready to trust your Divine CEO? Are you ready to align with His vision?

With God's guidance, I created ViaRayma™ as a practical, new way of practicing medicine — a way where Spirit and science are equally integrated and balanced. The 7 Alignments are the foundational basis for this approach to be effective. They allow you to embrace the work style your Divine CEO is asking you to embrace.

The ViaRayma Approach is how you now practice medicine as a Medical Intercessor, an upgrade to the authority already granted to you by your white coat. And this is just the foundational beginning. There is so much more to learn for even greater results. Become a ViaRayma Practitioner today! Check out the ad in the back of this book for more information.

Wherever your next steps take you, I pray for you to receive the guidance in this book, inspired by God, and for you to have a joyful, easy, light, and purpose-filled vocation in medicine. The world needs you!

Now that you have completed the 7 Alignments to bring you back to God, I encourage you to join the ViaRayma community of like-minded medical professionals walking the same transformative journey toward the impact that God is calling you to embrace as a Medical Intercessor. And keep returning to this book and the 7 Alignments Supplemental Content often, allowing the exercises to realign you with God's beautiful plan for your life and your practice. Let's create a White Coat Revival!

WhiteCoatRevival.com

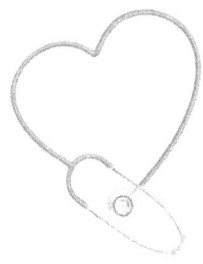

ENDNOTES

1   Dr. Caroline Leaf, Switch on Your Brain (Baker Publishing Group, 2013).

2   DW Baker, "Trust in Health Care in the Time of COVID-19," JAMA, 2020;324(23):2373—2375; and RH Perlis, K Ognyanova, A Uslu, Trujillo K Lunz, M Santillana, JN Druckman, MA Baum, and D Lazer, "Trust in Physicians and Hospitals During the COVID-19 Pandemic in a 50-State Survey of US Adults, JAMA Network Open 7, no. 7 (2024), doi: 10.1001/jamanetworkopen.

3   Yvette Brazier and Daniel Murrell, "What Is Ancient Greek Medicine?" Medical News Today, November 9, 2018, https://www.medicalnewstoday.com/articles/323596.

4   Dan Sullivan, Who Not How: The Formula to Achieve Bigger Goals Through Accelerating Teamwork (Hay House Business, 2020).

5   Steve Corn, "Jewish Educational System," November 1, 2010, https://stevecorn.com/2010/11/01/jewish-educational-system/.

6   "State of the U.S. Health Care Workforce, 2024," Health Resources & Services Administration, November 2024, https://bhw.hrsa.gov/sites/default/files/

bureau-health-workforce/state-of-the-health-workforce-report-2024.pdf.

7 State of the U.S. Health Care Workforce, 2024.

8 John Matheson, "Physician Suicide," American College of Emergency Physicians, accessed July 25, 2025, https://www.acep.org/life-as-a-physician/wellness/wellness/wellness-week-articles/physician-suicide.

9 Courses are available at ViaRayma.com, "Join Our Community," as of November 11, 2025.

10 Beth Powell, God Talks Mission Impossible event, San Diego, California July 13, 2025.

11 God Talks, Wisdom for Business event, Scottsdale, Arizona February 15–17, 2024

12 Andrew Wommack, Spirit, Soul and Body (Harrison House Publishers, 2010).

13 Merriam-Webster Dictionary, "faith," accessed July 29, 2025, https://www.merriam-webster.com/dictionary/faith.

14 John G. Lake Ministries, accessed July 28, 2025, https://www.jglm.org/about-jglm/.

15 Andrew Wommack, The Power of Imagination (Harrison House Publishers, 2019).

16 "Healing in the Book of Luke," Theology of Work Project, accessed July 26, 2025, https://www.theologyofwork.org/new-testament/luke/healing-luke/#:~:text=In%20Jesus'%20day%2C%20as%20now,demonized%2C%20and%20wounded.%E2%80%9D%5B.

17 Daniel D. Isgrigg, "The ORU Healing Hands," 2025, https://danieldisgrigg.com/2025/04/26/the-oru-healing-hands/.

18 "A Supernatural Vision: Mayo Clinic," Kairos Ministries, December 3, 2020, https://kairosmin.org/2020/12/03/a-supernatural-vision-mayo-clinic/.

19 Mark Bowles, "Our Healing Mission: Saint Francis
    Hospital and Medical Center," 2003, https://www.aca-
    demia.edu/4674033/Our_Healing_Mission_Saint_Francis_
    Hospital_and_Medical_Center?utm_source=chatgpt.
    com#loswp-work-container.

20 "John Alexander Dowe: The Healing Apostle," Reach the
    Nations Kingdom College, accessed July 28, 2025, http://
    www.rtnkc.org/pages.asp?pageid=114247.

21 "John G. Lake," Wikipedia, accessed July 26, 2025, https://
    en.wikipedia.org/wiki/John_G._Lake; also, "About John
    G. Lake, John G. Lake Ministries, accessed July 31, 2025,
    https://www.jglm.org/john-g-lake/.

22 Alyssa Roat, "What Is Agape Love? Bible Meaning and
    Examples," Christianity.com, May 28, 2025, https://www.
    christianity.com/wiki/christian-terms/what-does-agape-
    love-really-mean-in-the-bible.html.

23 Ed Rush, "Masterclass Live Recording," March 2024,
    Miramar Air Base, San Diego, CA.

24 Dallas Jenkins, The Chosen, television series, 5&2 Studios,
    December 24, 2017–present.

25 Joseph Z, God Talks Impossible event, San Diego, CA July
    13, 2025.

26 https://www.heartmath.com/science/

27 Illustration is from Ed Rush, various 2025 God Talks pre-
    sentations; godtalks.com, used with permission.

28 Brian Heasley, Be Still: A Simple Guide to Quiet Times
    (NavPress, 2023).

29 Chrissy Warrilow, "Solved: The Mystery of
    Double Rainbows," The Weather Channel, August
    27, 2014, https://weather.com/science/news/
    skywatching-double-rainbow-20130513.

30 Mark E. Moore, Quest 52: A Fifteen-Minute-a-Day
    Yearlong Pursuit of Jesus (Waterbrook, 2021).

31 F.F. Bosworth, Christ the Healer, (F.H. Revell Company, 1974)

32 Andrew Wommack, God Wants You Well: What the Bible Really Says About Walking in Divine Healing (Harrison House Publishers, 2009).

33 Global Celebrations, accessed July 26, 2025, https://www.globalcelebration.com/.

34 Kenneth E. Hagin, The Believer's Authority (Faith Library Publications, 1986).by Kenneth E. Hagin (https://a.co/d/aSp7WZ4

35 Goodreads, accessed July 26, 2025, https://www.goodreads.com/quotes/30608-i-m-a-little-pencil-in-the-hand-of-a-writing.

36 Elizabeth Vaughan, An Instrument in God's Hand: An Eye Surgeon's Discovery of The Miraculous (McDougal Publishing Company, 2018).

37 The Christian Broadcasting Network, "How a Little Boy's Brain Tumor Miracle Transformed Ben Carson's View of God." August 26, 2018. https://cbn.com/news/politics/how-little-boys-brain-tumor-miracle-transformed-ben-carsons-view-god

38 Personal communication, Heidi Reid, February 10, 2025

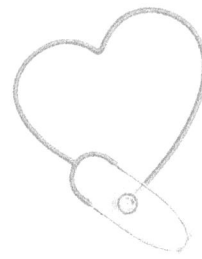

ACKNOWLEDGEMENTS

THANK YOU!

Thank you for reading my book and for joining me in changing the medical landscape, bringing hope and healing to this world as God originally designed. Thank you in advance for your obedience to God in flowing the love of Christ to your patients!

A big thank you to Nicole Gebhardt and her incredible Niche Press team for creating such a powerful transformation within me throughout the writing and publication process of the book. The inner journey was life-changing! Even as someone who's not a natural writer, I was able to bring to life the ideas and visions that were swirling inside my head. I'm beyond grateful for the way you all helped me give birth to this book that has the potential to transform many lives. It has truly been an amazing journey, and I couldn't have done it without you! If you ever desire to write a transformational book, be sure to connect with Niche Press.

Additionally, I want to give an extra thank you to Melanie, also with Niche Press, for the countless hours (months) she dedicated to assisting me with the authoring of this book. Thank God for her, so you all could enjoy reading it.

Thank you to the many family members and friends who helped shape, edit, and elevate this book into its finished form.

Thank you to my amazing husband and children, who stepped up throughout the many months I was submerged in the writing and editing of this book. I am beyond blessed to have your love and support!

And I want to especially thank all of the amazing authors and speakers who poured their hearts and souls into unpacking and teaching the New Covenant way of living that is so beautifully expressed in scripture. Your God-given understanding and wisdom have unlocked a profound power and authority for those who believe. Your wisdom and inspiration have shaped me greatly! I am forever transformed!

Thank you, Jesus! Thank you for choosing me to partner with you in writing this love letter to your children!

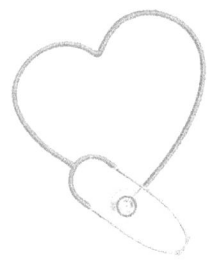

ABOUT THE AUTHOR

Marilyn Kaminski is the visionary founder of ViaRayma™, a movement revolutionizing healthcare through the collaboration of the Holy Spirit and science.

After months of visions, dreams, and downloads from God, she received a revelation from Him that healthcare professionals are called to more than just science-based medicine; they are called to bring complete healing by partnering with the Great Physician.

She has an advanced understanding of how to prepare your vessel and tap into the power created by your partnership with Christ, which has equipped many to reignite their purpose, unleash the power within them, and substantially transform patient outcomes.

With more than two decades of experience as an innovative medical professional — from Marilyn's early days as a nursing student to transitioning into sports medicine as a Licensed Certified Athletic Trainer, working in emergency sports medicine and injury prevention, to running her own independent clinic — she has always pursued healing beyond the limits of traditional practice.

Marilyn is known not only for her expertise but also for her bold faith, vibrant joy, and dynamic presence. When she speaks, she carries a contagious love and authority that captivates rooms and awakens the call of God within others. She dares providers to go beyond diagnosis and treatment, step into their true spiritual authority, and release miraculous healing. Her authenticity and servant's heart — marked by a love to serve without guile or ulterior motive — make her a powerful voice of hope and transformation in healthcare today.

Out of her passion to restore both providers and patients, Marilyn discovered the 7 Alignments™ necessary to reignite purpose, power, and patient outcomes, equipping you by blending clinical excellence with spiritual alignment.

Marilyn and her husband, Dave, are Kingdom-driven leaders in business and life, thoroughly enjoying raising their loving and energetic children, and often retreating to the mountains where their family finds refreshment and adventure.

CONTACT

Website: WhiteCoatRevival.com
Email: info@WhiteCoatRevival.com
LinkedIn: LinkedIn.com/In/MarilynHintz
Social: Facebook.com/ViaRayma and
Instagram.com/ViaRayma

ACCESS YOUR FREE
7 ALIGNMENTS™
SUPPLEMENTAL CONTENT

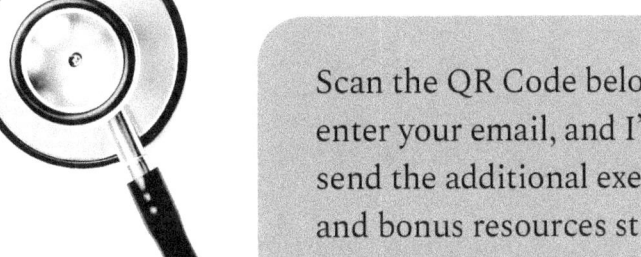

This book is designed with **alignment exercises** so you can pause and **realign** to optimize **your transformation** as you read.

Scan the QR Code below, enter your email, and I'll send the additional exercises and bonus resources straight to your inbox.

WhiteCoatRevival.com/bonus

Join the
ViaRayma
Community!

Join us in the **White Coat Revival** equipping you to be a purposeful and powerful Medical Intercessor!

Join like-minded individuals bringing heaven here on earth!

Become a Distinguished ViaRayma Practitioner

WhiteCoatRevival.com

Credentialing Courses Available!

Distinguish yourself as a practitioner who stands in the center of **Spirit** and **science**.

Help patients locate you. They have longed for this type of medicine for a long time!

HAS THIS BOOK
RESONATED WITH YOU?

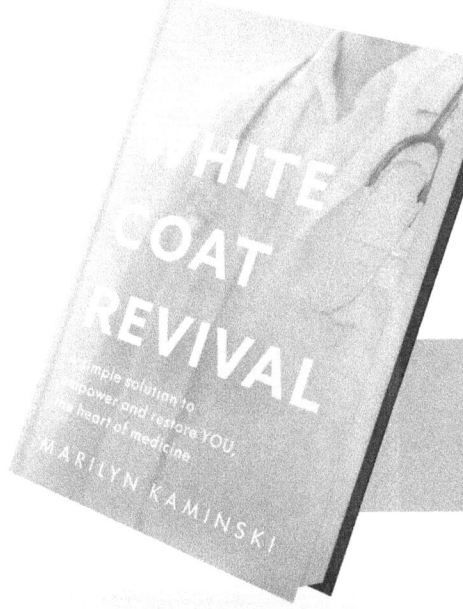

Have you felt the
immense power it
holds to transform
the **medical world**
as we know it?

**Imagine the ripple
effect this knowledge
could create!**

HIRE MARILYN AS A MENTOR

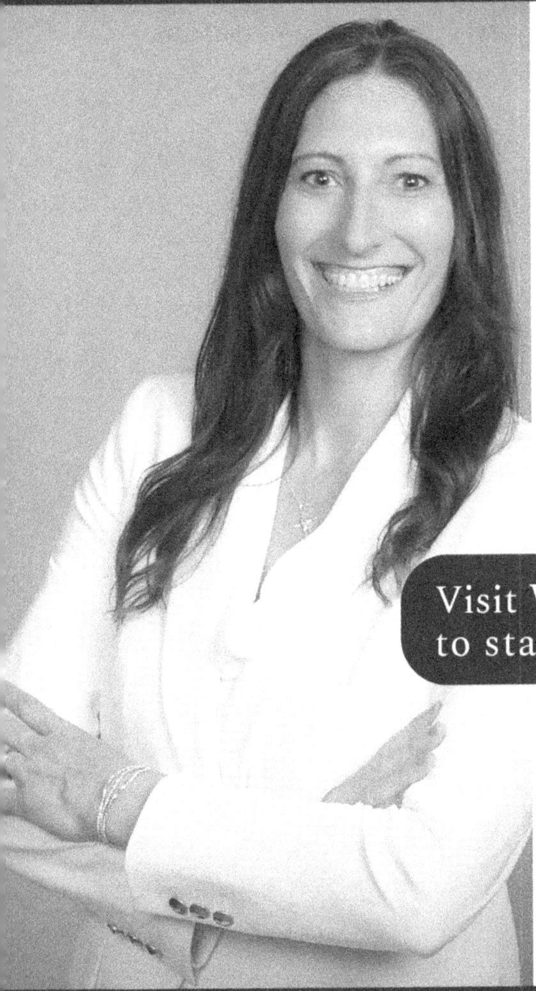

White Coat Revival offers incredible guidance to align with your purpose. But to truly leap into your higher calling as a Medical Intercessor, **partnering with a mentor can accelerate your journey.**

If you're ready to **fully align your profession with God's vision,** hire Marilyn as your professional mentor today.

Visit **WhiteCoatRevival.com** to start your transformation.

66 *There is no mentor like Marilyn. She brings a depth of wisdom in medicine and God I've never encountered. Her mentorship restored my family and reignited my calling beyond what I thought was possible.* 99

— Dr. Aister

Want to hire MARILYN to SPEAK at your next EVENT or PODCAST?

Transcend your event with Marilyn's captivating presence, energy and profound understanding of living aligned with God.

*She'll **inspire and empower** your **medical community** like never before!*